A Portrait of Breast Cancer

EXPRESSIONS IN WORDS AND ART

William D. Smith, PhD
Editor

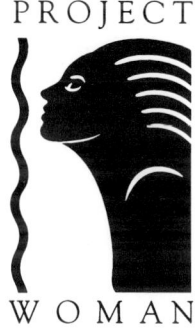

PROJECT

WOMAN

Published by
PROJECT WOMAN™
American Cancer Society
Oklahoma City, Oklahoma

A Portrait of Breast Cancer

EXPRESSIONS IN WORDS AND ART

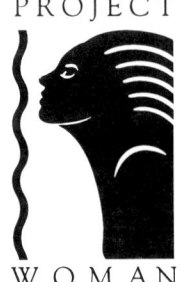

PROJECT

WOMAN

ISBN#[HC]: 0-9655886-0-2
[PB]: 0-9655886-1-0
PREVIOUSLY:
ISBN#[HC]: 0-927562-21-9
[PB]: 0-927562-19-7

Library of Congress Catalog
Number 96-06943

Published and distributed by
Project Woman™
American Cancer Society
Oklahoma City, Oklahoma

Printed by
Globe Color Press, Inc.
Oklahoma City, Oklahoma

Cover design by Rod Russell
in collaboration with Project Woman
Book Committee

Cover art, entitled *Another Healing
Revisited*, sculpture by Val Ray,
Oklahoma City, Oklahoma
(see page 99)

Editor
William D. Smith, PhD

**Project Woman™
Book Committee**
*Roseanna D. Smith, Chair
Dena Burton
Debbie Clark
Gay Conner
Melissa Craft
Paula Fulton
Terry Gonsoulin
Nancy Hane
Gennie Johnson
Pat Lynn Moses
Noel Tyler*

**American Cancer Society
Oklahoma Staff**
*Carrie Mitchell
Joy Stewart*

National Staff
*Beverly Greene
Janet Parrinello
Rod Russell
Kathy Tucker*

Special Thanks to
*Theresa Clark
Jennifer Deatsch
Sherry Fair
Laura Hoover Hughes
Deborah J. McKinley
Wanda Scott
Lee Allan Smith*

Foreword

Cathy Keating
First Lady of Oklahoma

The Project Woman Committee of the American Cancer Society has published *A Portrait of Breast Cancer* to honor and memorialize women who have had breast cancer. This book represents women whose stories will move and inspire you. The words and art express eloquently the experience of breast cancer as seen through the eyes, hearts, bodies and souls of those who have been there.

The women honored herein have their roots in the state of Oklahoma, but their personal accounts reflect the experiences of thousands of women and their families across our land who have confronted this disease: their shock and fear at discovering it, their rugged determination to face it and conquer it, their wit and wisdom in the midst of uncertainties, their reaching out to others for support and returning it in full measure, and their indelible faith and stabilizing outlook on life. It is an honor that we can pay tribute to them in this way.

But finally, this book is also a reminder—a reminder that lives continue to be threatened by this disease. All women are at risk and our hope is that *A Portrait of Breast Cancer* will encourage them to take charge of their lives by doing timely breast self examinations, and by seeking physicians' examinations and mammograms consistent with recommended guidelines. Advancements in research are promising. We must all dedicate ourselves to education and awareness so that this dreadful disease may soon be eradicated. That is the purpose of this book. That is our challenge!

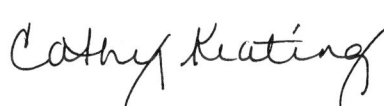

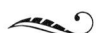
Art

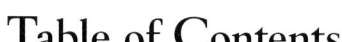

Table of Contents

Prologue

This is the kind of book I wanted to read when I learned that I had breast cancer. I clearly remember the time following my diagnosis. My husband and I would sit up in bed every night surrounded by stacks of books and materials about breast cancer as we frantically sought to learn as much as we could as fast as we could. We must have read hundreds of them, but what I was really looking for were the words of other women who had experienced what I was going through at that moment. I wanted to know what they thought, how they felt, how they managed their lives through this nightmare. I knew I could get answers to the medical questions from my physicians and from the piles of books in front of me. But what I wanted most was to hear the voice of someone who had been there.

All of us who have had breast cancer share the need for understanding what it is all about. It is that very need from which this book was born. It gives us a picture of the breast cancer experience through the eyes of the women themselves, their children, husbands, sisters, mothers, nieces, and other relatives and friends. It portrays in words and art the stories of young women who feared they would never have children or might never be able to nurse a child with a remaining breast. It reveals the emotions of eight-year-old children whose mothers grappled with the disease, and of eighty-year-old women who had to deal with it.

This is a book about courage—courage that many of us never realized we had: courage to face surgery perhaps for the first time; courage to take on the fear of the unknown; courage to appear in public or even in front of our families, friends and associates after losing breasts, hair and feminine grace—those things that once defined us, enhanced our self-image and helped us to face others; courage to ask hard questions and to be braced for tougher answers; courage to face frightening options that our very lives might depend on.

This is a book about sharing—the sharing of common experiences, of lessons learned; sharing in the hope that our stories may bring comfort, reassurance and peace to another who is in pain; sharing to find some deeper understanding of a life-altering event; sharing in order to nourish the healing process. The very act of creating the words and drawing the pictures promotes healing. The sculpture portrayed on the cover of this book, and entitled *"Another Healing Revisited,"* is symbolic of the healing that occurs when you express in words or art what you experience in facing a traumatic event like breast cancer. This book is an anthology of such experiences. The dream of *Project Woman* would be to encourage you to *tell your story*—keep a diary, write a poem, record a daily log of what happens and how you feel. And, we trust that reading the stories and seeing the pictures may serve as a balm to others and give hope to all of us as we make our journey together.

Roseanna D. Smith

Roseanna D. Smith, Chair
Project Woman Book Committee

Project Woman Book Committee

Roseanna D. Smith, Chair

Dena Burton

Debbie Clark

Gay Conner

Melissa Craft

Paula Fulton

Terry Gonsoulin

Nancy Hane

Gennie Johnson

Carrie Mitchell

Pat Lynn Moses

Joy Stewart

Noel Tyler

William D. Smith, Editor

Editor's Notes

In 1995, *Project Woman* Committee launched its search throughout the state of Oklahoma for women who have encountered breast cancer. *Phase I* of the project was a photographic exhibit of women who were nominated, reviewed, and selected by the Committee; *Phase II* is this book of writings and art by nominees who likewise were reviewed and selected by the Committee. [A more complete description of the origins and mission of *Project Woman* can be found in the Epilogue of this book.] Hundreds of nominees were received for both parts of the project. The forms for each applicant included biographical information, descriptions of the nominee with respect to age, facts about her diagnosis and current breast cancer status, her life's work and interests, plus authorization for use of materials and a release form for signature. It is pertinent to note here that the information found in this publication is based on facts presented at the time of the application. All biographical information, art and textual materials which appear in this book required signed releases by the applicant and/or person nominating that individual. In addition, textual materials were edited for length and clarity and then released with approval by signature of the applicant and/or person nominating that individual.

A final word. As editor of this book, I must applaud the members of the Project Woman Book Committee for the competent, collaborative and compassionate way they approached and completed this challenging task. It was a labor of love. The majority are themselves survivors of breast cancer and a living testament to the values revealed in this book. Their foremost wish was to remember and honor with distinction their fellow sojourners. They did so with great respect and admiration. But the greater acclaim, of course, belongs to the women whose stories and pictures you are about to see and the thousands of others whom they represent. We salute them.

1
Finding It and Facing It
"This can't be!"

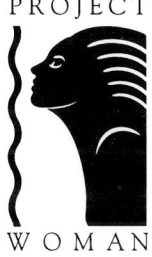

1
Finding It and Facing It
"This can't be!"

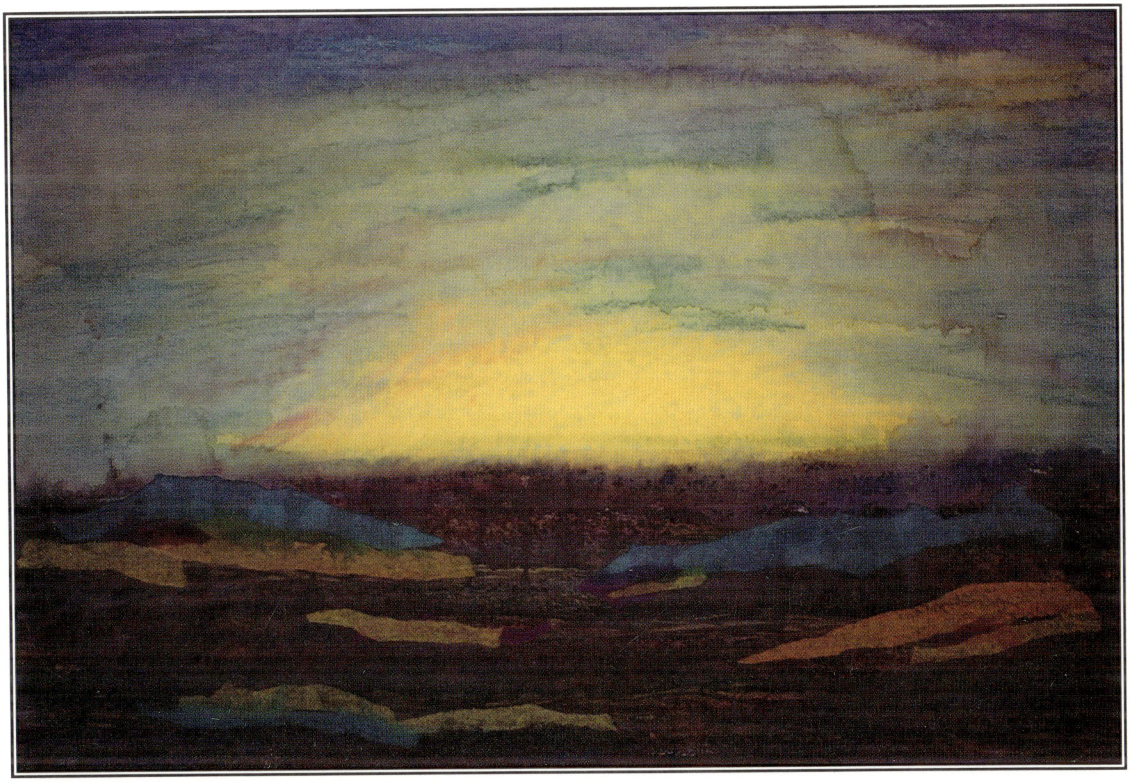

"Sunrise? Sunset?"   Pat Lynn Moses

Pat Lynn Moses, a breast cancer survivor, completed this mixed media piece while undergoing chemotherapy. The art expressed her questions: "Is this the end of my life, or might it be a new beginning?" Pat Lynn's story is on pages 60-61. Please note also that Pat Lynn, an Art Therapist, created and initialed (PLM) other pieces of line art in this book. She was instrumental as well in coordinating the art work that is integral to this publication.

This Can't Be!
Violet Lee Hunter

I had thought about the day I would die. I would be very old and tired, with wrinkles. My children would be all grown and gray. My grandchildren would be graduated from college and jumping into the real world. I had taken life for granted; planned everything out just the way I wanted it to be. Then, on a cold January day in 1990, I went to my Ob/Gyn for a routine exam. It was time for my annual Pap smear. I was really stressed out coping with the death of my father four months prior and the death of my mother four months before that.

Before going to the doctor, I had noticed my left breast was sporting a lump. There was no pain, nothing abnormal about it; I just figured it was a swollen gland. My Ob/Gyn insisted that I see a surgeon. When the surgeon aspirated the breast and nothing came out, I became frantic! Is this it? This can't be! Death at 35? My mind raced to the inevitable as I saw flashbacks of TV commercials about the odds of getting breast cancer and the statistics on deaths from breast cancer. I felt alone. I couldn't tell my parents; they were now gone. Then I thought, I'm just jumping the gun, maybe it's nothing. Sleep became foreign to me; I would doze off only to wake up feeling anxious.

To be sure, a biopsy was taken. As the doctor approached me, I had this look of horror on my face. She then whispered to me the words that changed by life: "Lee, I am so sorry, but the tumor in your breast is malignant and I suggest the entire breast be removed."

That was five years ago. I am now approaching my sixth year of survival. Instead of concentrating on where I want to be years from now, I live each day as it comes and know there is a tomorrow.

Violet Lee Hunter, age 41, of Oklahoma City. Lee is a 14-year employee with the V.A. Medical Center in Oklahoma City, serving as program assistant to the chief of police and security service. She was diagnosed at age 35, and is now an active grandmother who enjoys public speaking and participating in annual softball classics. Lee is also a member of Reach to Recovery and a volunteer for the National Black Women Health Survey in Boston, Massachusetts.

Sandy's Journal
Sandy Brown

Sept. / 16:

   I accidently laid my hand over some type of lump in my right breast. I can't be sure how long its been there, since I've never done self exams. My doctor told me to, especially since I'm over 50, but breast cancer doesn't run in my family. I've never even had a mammogram. Guess I better have one now.

Oct. / 12:

   Finally had time to have that mammogram. The doctor was so concerned by what she found, she insisted I make an appointment with a surgeon before leaving her office. Doctors can be such alarmists. This is nothing to worry about. I am a very healthy woman.

Oct. / 16:

   The surgeon says I need a biopsy. No big deal. It's an outpatient procedure that will only take a few hours, if it isn't cancer. It won't be.

Oct / 18:

   A friend will drop me off at the hospital and pick me up this afternoon. I'll be glad when this is over so I can go on with my life!

Oct / 25:

   Funny how a week can feel like a year. I've been in a dream world since I last wrote. A nightmare to be more accurate. It was cancer. How can this be happening to me? I still feel dazed. Like I'm watching someone else's life from a distance. It had not spread to my lymph nodes. What are lymph nodes? Twenty-two of mine were removed. How many do I've left? Is it enough? They said I chose to have a lumpectomy rather than a mastectomy and that I'm lucky because a few years ago I would not have had the choice. I don't feel lucky. I don't even remember making the decision. What if I was wrong? God help me. Anyway, I'm home. There is a tube running from my breast to a neat little plastic bag taped to my waist so the incision can drain. I have to do a few exercises so I won't permamently lose arm motion. Like I said, a nightmare.

Nov./10

Got the drain out today. Next comes a visit with an oncologist.

Nov./15

The oncologist said I need chemotherapy. I broke down sobbing ~ my first tears since this whole thing began. The possibility of losing my hair took me over the edge. First I have cancer. Now I might be bald. Too many new experiences for this gal. I have my first of six doses next week. After the third one, I start seven weeks of daily radiation therapy. And to think I quit smoking so I wouldn't poison my body.

April /26

In the last seven months I've survived breast cancer and more importantly, its treatment. All of my priorities have shifted. I'm more careful about how I treat people and what I let upset me. Although I will always take good care of my body, I've seen its temporal nature. I'm more concerned about my spirit these days. I think I'll go ahead and take that trip to Yellowstone.

Sandy Brown, age 55, of Oklahoma City. Sandy, who was diagnosed at age 51, worked for United Parcel Service until six months after her diagnosis. She took disability, followed by early retirement. At present she is involved in several areas of volunteer work. Her main enjoyment comes from working with individuals who are attempting to improve the quality of their lives. (Please note that the calligraphy was created by Sandy's friend, Roseanna Smith.)

Unexpected Visitor
Ruth Pratt

Cancer was not something I thought about or feared in a personal way. I knew the life stories of my grandmothers, my mother, all my sisters, aunts, cousins, nieces and my own daughter. Not one of them had cancer of any kind.

Then, after a routine physical exam which included a mammogram, the radiologist called me in to look at the x-rays. He pointed to an area which looked like a little bundle of fibers. He referred to it as a "worrisome spot" and insisted that I have a biopsy immediately. One week later, I did. After the procedure was completed, I was brought back to my hospital room, nauseous and dizzy. Soon my good doctor came in and stood quietly by my bed. I asked if he had the report yet. He said, "Yes. It's cancer." Instantly I heard myself blurt out in a strong voice, "That makes me so mad! WELL, I JUST REFUSE TO HAVE IT!!" After a hurried conference with my husband in the hallway outside my room, the doctor asked that I come to his office two days later to check the biopsy incision, at which time we would talk about the cancer.

During that appointment, he said in a gentle way, "I don't know just what you want from me." I told him that I would like for him to tell me what my options were, and then I could decide what I would do. To his credit, he did exactly that without trying to coerce me. As he described the details of a mastectomy, I suddenly felt sick and the floor began spinning around and around. I quickly said, "I am not going to have that operation. What else is there?" He then told me of a procedure called a lumpectomy, which removes only the portion of the breast containing the cancer. I had not known much about it until then, but it sounded right for me. We scheduled the surgery for one week from that very day. During the next several days, my husband and I devoured every piece of information we could find about breast cancer and what needed to be done.

Happily, the surgery was a complete success! At no time during the whole experience did I think of myself as "sick." My point of view was that my breast had a small cancer; I did not. Of the many deep lessons I gained from this experience, the more important ones are that we can have access to love and strength through our attitudes, faith and prayers, and a God-given mind to make our own decisions. Had I skipped the mammogram that year, I might be telling a very different story—or none at all!

Ruth Pratt, age 76, of Tulsa. Submitted by her daughter, Peggy Ann Pratt. Ruth, diagnosed at age 70, has spent "half a century" as a wife, mother, homemaker, artist and an "unpaid minister of upliftment" to friends and family all over the United States. Peggy says her mother embodies all the special traits of "good mothering," including honesty, unconditional love, wise boundaries, respect, and really being with a person "in the moment."

Stunned
Muriel Wallace

I woke up on Friday morning and felt something odd in my breast. I told my husband Russell about it. During my dental appointment, I asked my dentist who he would recommend if he'd just learned that his wife had a lump in her breast. He sent me down the hall to a colleague. After a needle biopsy and x-rays, they told me the lump needed to come out. On the way to surgery, I told the doctor to do whatever was necessary if it was malignant. Back in my room, I woke up to find my entire right breast gone. I was stunned to be without my breast. Even though I lost my father, brother and a sister to cancer, I've never felt that it would get me.

Muriel Wallace, age 82, of Ponca City, as dictated to her daughter, Audrey Barr. Muriel, a homemaker and mother, was diagnosed at age 62. She has served as president of the local American Association of Retired Persons, delivered Mobile Meals, and she visits local nursing homes twice weekly.

Everything Happened So Fast
Joanne Abernathy

Joanne Abernathy was 49 when she was told she had breast cancer. Her sister also had breast cancer at the same age and survived that disease, but died later of cervical cancer. Joanne underwent a mammogram and later got a call from one of her doctor's associates. "He told me, 'We just got the results of your mammogram and we think it's cancer'—just like that." She was scheduled for immediate surgery. "There I am in the hospital for surgery. My husband wasn't even home from work. Everything happened so fast." Joanne's tumor was found to be malignant and cancer was found in two of her lymph nodes. She underwent a mastectomy, radiation, and chemotherapy treatments. She has been a cancer survivor for 13 years. "Luckily, I'm still here to tell about it," she says.

Joanne Abernathy, age 62, of Poteau. Excerpts from an article written by Fran Johnson, Heavener Ledger, and submitted by Dee Ann Dickerson, Chair of the LeFlore County Women's Health Coalition in Poteau, Oklahoma. Joanne is a retired music instructor. She told her story of courage at the Women's Health Forum in Poteau, April 1, 1995.

A Second Chance
Lynne Thompson

"We need you to come in for some magnifications." It was a cold, cloudy March morning when I got that call. I remember shaking uncontrollably for about a minute. I worked in a school for handicapped children; so I got a grip and went on with the day's activities.

I had just had my mammogram the previous day. It was the first one in five years. My mother had one every year and insisted I do the same; she would pay for it. But I said, "Mother, I'm not even 40 yet and I don't need a mammogram every year." The fact is that I had found a lump in the outer quadrant of my left breast six months earlier, but I felt very confident it was not cancerous because there was no history of breast cancer in my family. This time, a bit self-consciously, I mentioned it to my gynecologist. He felt confident it was fibrocystic disease but encouraged me to have the mammogram.

That night I could not sleep. I had run the gamut of emotions—disbelief, shock, and feeling I had been hit by a Mack truck. And boy was I anxious! My mind raced with the thought of going for a second opinion, and then saying, "No, no, go with the surgery and get it over with!"

I prayed to God to please help me decide what to do. Suddenly the most peaceful calm came over me. I knew in that instant that I would go with the surgery and get on with my life. My husband sensed my restlessness and stroked my cheek. I told him what had just happened and then felt the tears rolling down his cheeks as he pulled me closer to him.

The surgery was performed on April 1. Upon waking, my first question to my husband was, "Did they take my breast?" He told me they did. From that moment I have looked straight ahead. I never saw myself as deformed or less than a woman. I never looked in the mirror, disgusted at what I saw. I was alive! I had been given a second chance.

Lynne Thompson, age 42, of Norman. Lynne works in the Norman Public School system, and has been a preschool director and a teacher's assistant. During University of Oklahoma football games, she offers day care services. Diagnosed at age 40, Lynne was captain of the Norman breast cancer support group's Relay for Life team for two years.

The Long Weekend
Lois Kennemer

I discovered the knot in my breast on Friday. I decided I would not say anything to anyone until Monday morning. Monday came. I told my husband; he called our daughter. The mammogram was very suspicious, so the doctor removed the knot. It was malignant. He removed the complete breast the next day.

When I was around other people in the hospital, it was okay; once I arrived home and looked in my mirror, it was different. My husband and I cried in each other's arms. I haven't cried about it since. I had reconstruction in August. Of course, it's not like what God gave me, but there is something there.

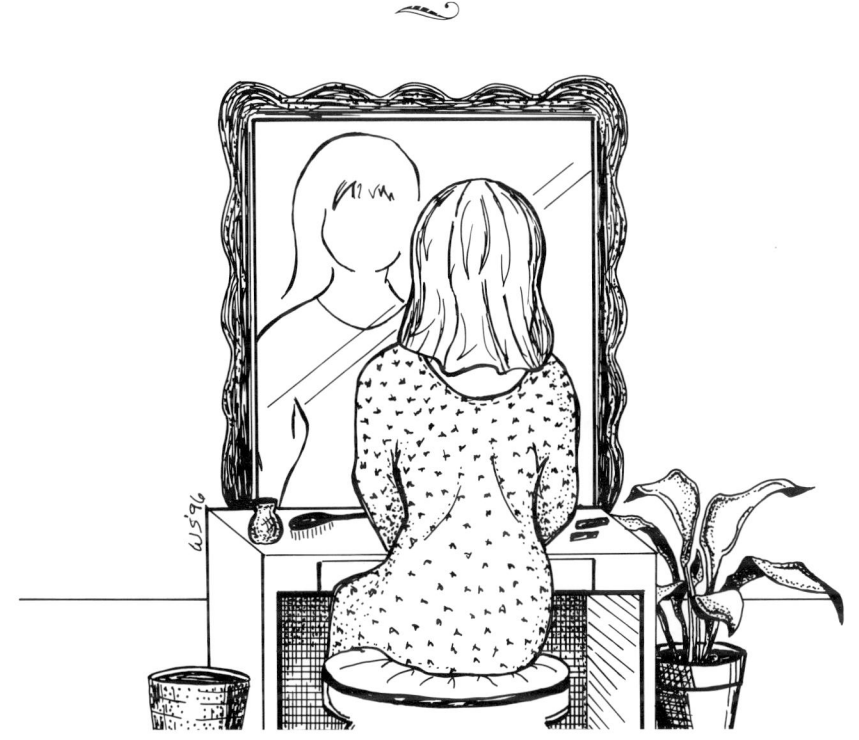

Lois Kennemer, age 61, of Dill City. Lois, a homemaker, wife, secretary, mother and grandmother, was diagnosed at age 48. She watched her two grandsons while their parents worked, loves her flowers and vegetable gardens, and spends her remaining time doing floral arrangements for family and friends.

The line art on this page, called "The Mirror," was drawn by Wanda Scott. Please note other pieces of art which she has created and initialed (WS) in this book. Wanda dedicates her artistic work in honor of her mother, Rachel Wade, who was diagnosed with breast cancer in 1993 at age 77 as a result of her first mammogram. Rachel is a cattle ranch owner, a mother, a grandmother and great-grandmother, and is a survivor! Wanda stated: "I now live with the knowledge that breast cancer is no respecter of persons. My participation in the production of this book is with the hope of educating women that early detection can save lives."

By Faith
Mary Pace Falling

My first thought was, "I'm going to die." As a nurse, I remembered patients and friends who had gone through disfiguring surgery, radiation and chemotherapy, only to have cancer return. The doctors told me to live one day at a time. Because of lymph node involvement, I was at high risk for recurrence. This left me feeling helpless, hopeless and very depressed.

Through my family, caring doctors and a local cancer support group, I overcame these feelings. I am living by faith, contributing where God can use me. Life can go on after a diagnosis of cancer.

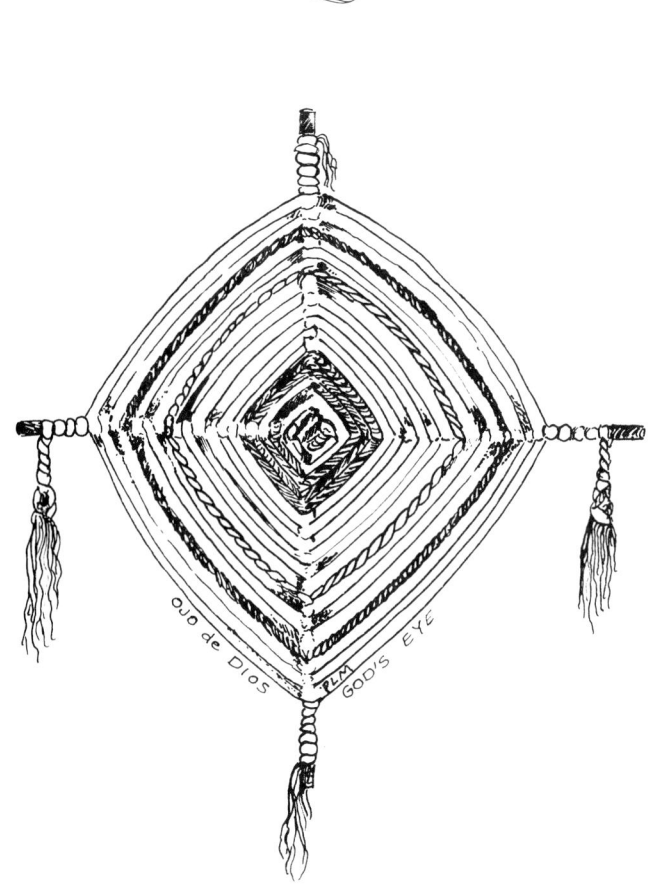

Mary Falling, age 56, of Tahlequah. Mary, a registered nurse, was diagnosed at age 52. She is co-director and founder of the Crisis Pregnancy Center of Tahlequah, a volunteer for Meals on Wheels and the American Red Cross, serves as an RN for her church camp, and participates as an RN on medical missions to Honduras.

A Discouraging Word
Mary Burchett

It was a busy time in January; so busy that I did not take time to call in for my yearly mammogram. I always have that done during the month of my birthday—that way I won't forget. But a hectic schedule caused me to wait until March. When I did call the doctor's office for the appointment, much to my surprise I was not able to get in until May.

When I finally went in, the technician who took my mammogram asked me to come back in for another one. I didn't think much about it; just figured I must have breathed or moved when they were taking the picture. Some time later, I got a call from the doctor's office. They wanted me to come back in for a consultation. I was rather surprised they had questions about the results of my mammogram. They had found a lump that looked "suspicious."

After talking with the doctors, one of them asked me if I would like to see the mammogram. I said yes. In the meantime I had picked up some pamphlets on breast cancer. I then realized that my x-ray and the pamphlet picture of a malignant tumor looked the same—not a lump but like little stars. I asked my husband on the way home if it looked malignant to him. He said, "Well, it could be, but let's just wait and see."

I had the surgery. In the recovery room afterwards, the surgeon told me that the lump was cancerous. While I was somewhat prepared for it, I was still quite disturbed. The word cancer is such a powerful and disheartening word! But it was detected early and removed quickly. And now, two years later, I am still cancer-free. There is hope—there is life.

Mary Burchett, age 57, of Midwest City. Mary was diagnosed at age 55. She is a pastor's wife, a mother and grandmother. She served as a part-time secretary at her husband's church, and loves to babysit her grandchildren. Mary is a member of the Midwest City Christian Women's Club and the Life Christian Center.

2
Any Color, Any Age
"It shows no prejudice."

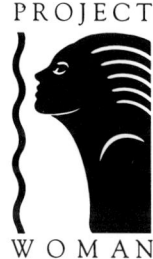

2
Any Color, Any Age
"It shows no prejudice."

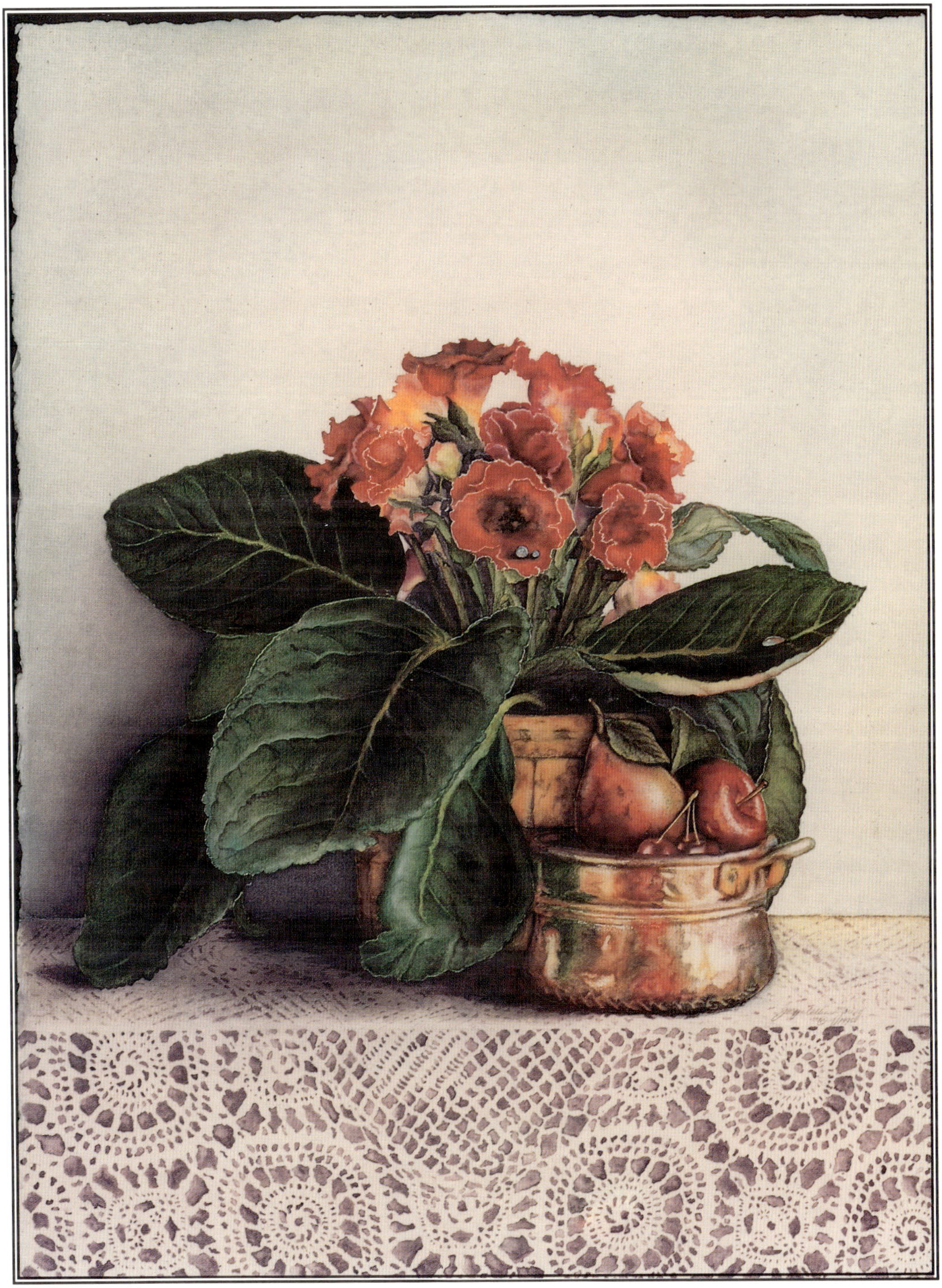

"Granma's Treasures"   Jacque Collins Young

Jacque Collins Young, a watercolor artist, is featured at the beginning of five chapters in this book: chapters 2, 3, 4, 5, and 7. This piece was done as a gift for her mother. Jacque's personal story as a breast cancer survivor is found on page 26.

Cancer Shows No Prejudice
Beatrice J. Samis

As one whose mother died of breast cancer, and a member of the Comanche tribe, I want to convince people that all races are susceptible to cancer. Cancer shows no prejudice! And, based upon my experiences as a volunteer for the American Cancer Society "Circle of Life" program, I want to teach the members of my community about the need for early detection. I learned that cancer is not a death sentence.

Beatrice Samis, age 62, of Cache. Beatrice was 56 when she was diagnosed and continues to volunteer time to educate others about breast cancer and how to deal with the experience. In addition to her work with the American Cancer Society, she works with children at her church. She also worked for 21 years for the Comanche tribe.

It Came Unexpectedly
Patricia Gutierrez Horner

In my case, cancer came unexpectedly. I don't have a single risk factor, but when one out of eight women in the U.S. may get breast cancer in their lifetime, I just believe it was my turn. Some have asked me how I've dealt with this ordeal. First, I had the deep conviction that God was watching over me. Second, I was fortunate to find a wonderful support group. Third, we haven't been alone. Family and friends have been a wonderful source of love and support.

Patricia Horner, age 38, of Poteau. Submitted by her friend, Carole Gill. Patricia, who has held various social service positions, was diagnosed at age 37. She has served as a vocational counselor, performed various services for the disabled, and has been a teacher. Her interests include teaching a Mexican cooking class, working for her church, and serving as a bilingual volunteer for the county health department.

Can't Always Trust the Statistics
Lisa A. Efaw

Diagnosed at age 27, I am an example of how early detection can help save a life from breast cancer. We cannot always trust statistics; younger women can and do get breast cancer. Everyone needs to know how to do self-examinations and how to trust their own instincts about their bodies. Also, women need to see positive life-continuing stories. Life does not have to end when you hear the word cancer. If you maintain a positive outlook and faith in God, you can beat it.

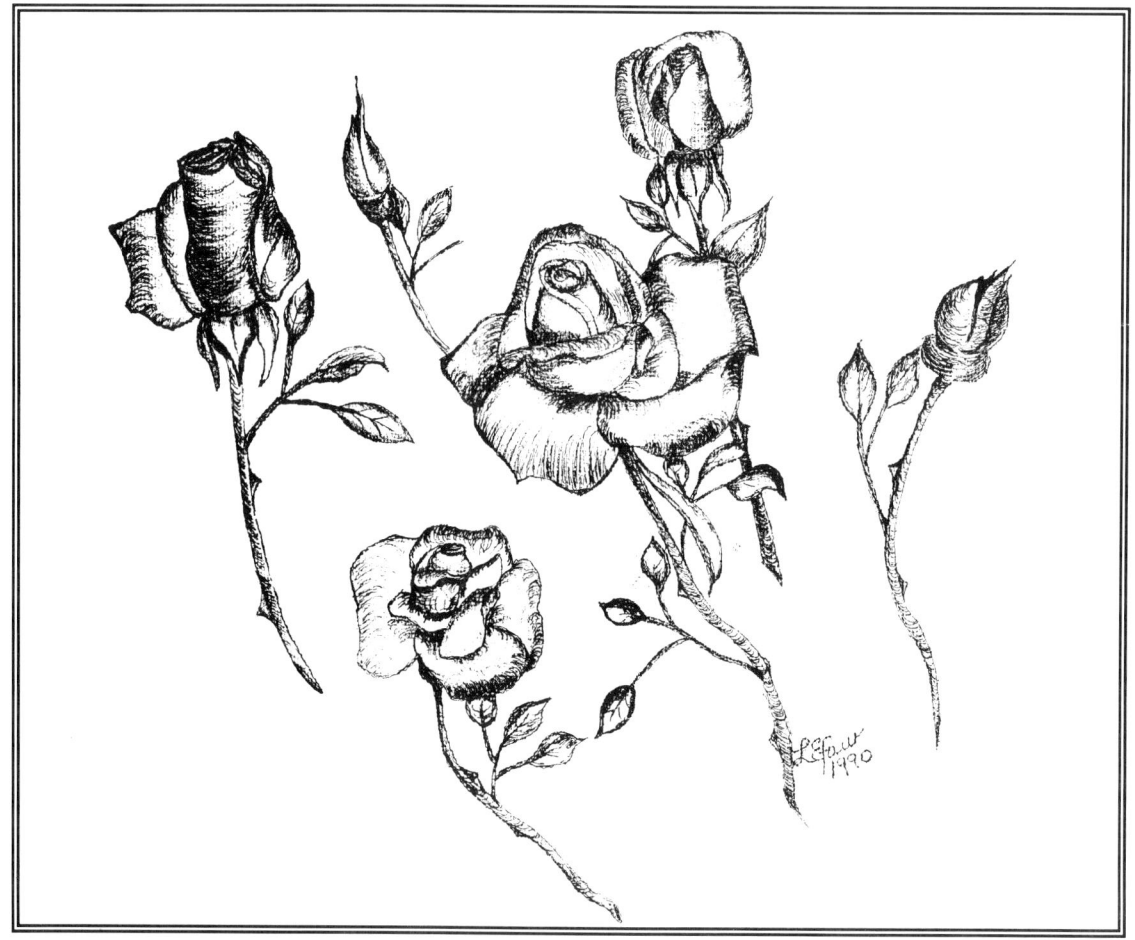

"Roses"

Lisa A. Efaw

Lisa Efaw, age 39, of Broken Arrow. Lisa dedicates this in memory of Mary Sippy, a friend who died of breast cancer in February 1993. Lisa is a PTA mom for two schools, a 4th grade Sunday school teacher, choir teacher, Reach to Recovery volunteer, and the coordinator of the CornerStone Mission of the First Baptist Church. It should be noted that Efaw contributed this piece of art, entitled "Roses."

My Life Line
Shawn Curtis

The mammogram showed a cancer growing behind the nipple of my right breast. A biopsy confirmed it. I felt sick, choking, gripping sick. I would have to have a mastectomy. My husband sat by my side and held my hand. I was 35, a wife and a mother of two boys, eight and five years old. And now cancer was invading my life.

Donald brought me home after the surgery. The hard part was bath time and seeing the bandage where my right breast had been. It was even harder, two days later, when the surgeon removed the bandages. There it was—the incision, the scar, the stitches. I started to cry and then my husband said, "Doctor, you did a good job. That is a very nice stitch up." It made me feel good. He did not have that "oh it's horrible looking" stare on his face. "I'm glad you're alive," he said. He made me feel good about myself.

It is seven months later and my scar is now called my life line. This is the spot where God pulled a deadly killer out of me. I have a second chance at life. I want young women to know that breast cancer needs to be taken seriously. This killer disease knows no age boundary. Breast cancer can happen to any woman.

Shawn Curtis, age 36, of Moore. Shawn spends most of her time looking after her children and helping her husband, Trooper Donald Curtis. A former horse trainer, she later became a banker before staying at home to be a full-time mother. If you ask Shawn what her "life work" is now, her answer is that it began again at age 35 when she was diagnosed with breast cancer.

I Never Thought
Sherry Ann Brulé

Speaking to the hospice organization about Sherry succumbing to breast cancer, Kris, her husband, said:

"I never thought she would die so young (age 38). I saw us growing old together, watching our grandchildren grow up. Cancer is not discriminating as to age or apparent good health. My wife was a healthy, attractive lady who was struck down because of breast cancer. As a teacher of journalism, she spent the best years of her life educating young minds. Through her story, she continues to educate society about the devastation caused by cancer. She has taught me courage, tenacity, and humor."

Comments by Kris Brulé, husband of Sherry Ann Brulé, of Edmond, who died at age 38. Includes excerpts from Kris' interview about the Brulé family's experiences as reported in the Mercy Health Center hospice publication, At Home. Sherry taught journalism at the Mayfield Junior High School, sponsoring the school newspaper and yearbook for 10 years. She was a gifted teacher, respected by students and teachers alike. In addition to her professional work, Sherry was a loving wife and mother and, as the most organized person Kris had ever met, she gave relentless time and energy to her family. According to Kris, "Sherry gave 100% to everything she did!"

Do Something Positive
Beth Snider

When I was diagnosed at age 32, I was younger than the average breast cancer patient. My sister also had breast cancer when she was 39 years old, and I've had two aunts and one cousin who had breast cancer as well. I am participating in a breast cancer project through the University of Oklahoma Health Sciences Center.

I also work as a volunteer for the American Cancer Society's Reach to Recovery program, and church and community activities, including Big Brothers/Big Sisters. Younger breast cancer patients need to see someone closer to their own age who has survived and returned to a healthy, active lifestyle. I believe that no matter what happens to us along life's highway, God gives us the opportunity to do something positive with the experience.

Beth Snider, age 37, of Woodward. Beth, a secretary, was diagnosed at age 32, but keeps an active life of community, church and civic duties. She is active in Big Brothers/Big Sisters, and loves rollerblading with her "Little Sister" in the organization.

So Alone
LaDonna Taylor

As I was drying off after my nightly shower, my hand felt a strange lump. At first I thought "oh no! I'm only 29 years old. I'm finally happy and married and have a two-year-old. It can't be cancer!" But it was. I had my right breast removed and then had chemotherapy once a week for a year.

I told my supervisor I would need to take off one hour every Thursday to go for treatments. He looked me straight in the eye and said, "Oh, you're going to milk this for all it's worth." I said, "What!" He said, "You're going to take advantage of this." I fired back, "You bet I will if there's a chance it will keep me alive." I went every Thursday. Sometimes on Fridays I felt so weak and tired I had to lean on the wall so I could make it through work. The trash can beside me became my best buddy.

Everything was going great until October, five years later. The big "C" reared its head again. I had to have a hysterectomy. I thought, I can handle this; it's not as bad as losing a breast. But the following year, I found another lump. This time I went in for the biopsy with the understanding that if it were cancerous, the surgeon would do the mastectomy at once. Yet, I was shocked and horrified when I awoke to discover that my left breast was gone. I just kept thinking there is no way a woman in her thirties could have cancer three times and lose both breasts. But it can happen and did.

My biggest problem is feeling so alone. It seems even your friends don't know what to say, so they don't say anything. Eventually, you never hear from them anymore. No one will ever know how it feels unless they have been through it. Live every day the best you can. Let people know you love them. Life is too short and you just never know what can happen.

LaDonna Taylor, age 35, of Midwest City. LaDonna worked in an automobile assembly plant for 14 years, retiring in 1993 after an injury to her left shoulder. Her right breast was diagnosed with cancer in 1989, and her left breast was diagnosed in 1995. She is active in the PTA and has been a homeroom mother for the past three years. She is involved in her church and in Helping Hands at Soldier Creek School.

It Can Happen to You
Sharon Fisher

Sharon has faced one adversity after another during the past eight years beginning with the removal of her colon in 1988, additional intestinal surgery in 1993 and breast cancer at age 34 in 1994. In spite of what for most would be a struggle beyond human endurance, she not only has survived but she serves as an inspiration to others by exhibiting strength, courage, and determination to achieve her life's goal of helping others through her medical training.

Sharon's experience underscores the fact that breast cancer is not limited to any specific age group. Breast cancer is being diagnosed in younger women in greater numbers than ever before. As Sharon says: "Every woman needs to maintain a regular routine of monthly breast self-examinations because you never think it's gonna happen to you!"

Sharon Fisher, age 35, of Oklahoma City. Submitted by her husband, Michael Fisher. Sharon was diagnosed with breast cancer at age 34, and has been employed as a clinical research coordinator in the Department of Urology at the University of Oklahoma Health Sciences Center for the past 10 years. She volunteered for the American Cancer Society's Oklahoma City Unit breast cancer hotline, and is a member of the Central Oklahoma Chapter of the Susan G. Komen Breast Cancer Foundation and is a volunteer for Race for the Cure. In spite of her own health situation, Sharon found time for others when she volunteered for the American Red Cross in the wake of the bombing of the Murrah Building in Oklahoma City, April 19, 1995.

Third Generation
Rebecca Day

Being diagnosed with breast cancer last year, right after my 36th birthday, was absolutely terrifying. I represent an age group of women who don't really worry about breast cancer. Many people think it happens only to older women. I am the third generation in my family to have breast cancer: my grandmother, my mother's sister, and now me. All of us are survivors. My biggest fear is that this "legacy" will be passed on to my two beautiful daughters.

Rebecca Day, age 37, of Owasso. Rebecca was diagnosed at age 36, and works in a family practice medical clinic. A wife and mother of three, Rebecca is a third generation breast cancer survivor in her family.

Any Little Illness Scares Me
Sandra Edwards

Sandra is a single mom with two children. Her family stands as a model for minority women to have mammograms on a regular basis.

Sandra fought through depression, determined not to let her illness change her life. She returned to her job full-time, and worked to make her life normal once more. However, it hasn't been easy, for breast cancer is a dominant factor in her family. Sandra's maternal aunt just completed her fifth year after a mastectomy; her mother had a mastectomy in June, 1955. Sandra was diagnosed with breast cancer in 1992 at age 35. This experience has brought the three of them closer together as they support each other.

Recently Sandra found a lump on her right breast. This one was benign. "Any little illness scares me," Sandra said, but she is determined not to let it get her down.

Sandra Edwards, age 38, of Tulsa. Submitted by her friend, Jerry Jones. Sandra, a hospital admissions representative, was diagnosed at age 35. A single mother of two, Sandra is a native Tulsan and studies with Jehovah's Witnesses Kingdom Hall.

Magic Colors
Jacque Collins Young

Magic colors—that's how Tulsa artist Jacque Collins Young views the world. As a child growing up on an Oklahoma farm, Jacque was fascinated by the magic of colors. Nature's kaleidoscope—sunlight dancing through vivid greens of trees, glorious red-gold and purple sunsets, Cerulean blue and thunderous blacks and grays of Oklahoma skies—bring strong influence to her watercolors. Casual interest became full-time dedication when a health crisis caused her to listen to her heart and pursue art more seriously.

I grew up on a dairy farm in Rogers County near Verdigris in a family of nine children. Our family is very close and our lives chock full of traditions. We are members of the Cherokee Indian Nation. Our extended family joyfully embraces 70–80 relatives. During my medical challenge in 1989, I had lots of time to think, pray, and find out the most important things in life. One of my strongest influences has always been my family, its heritage and traditions. I hope other women can look at life and receive encouragement. Believe in yourself and welcome the love, support, and prayers of your family and friends.

Jacque Collins Young, age 51, of Tulsa. Jacque, a wife, mother, homemaker, and watercolor artist, was diagnosed at age 45. As a member of the Cherokee Indian Nation and in a close knit family, Jacque, her mother and sisters recently completed a family cookbook and memory book, titled "A Little Bit of This & That." Two years in the making, this book will serve as a family keepsake to be passed down from generation to generation.

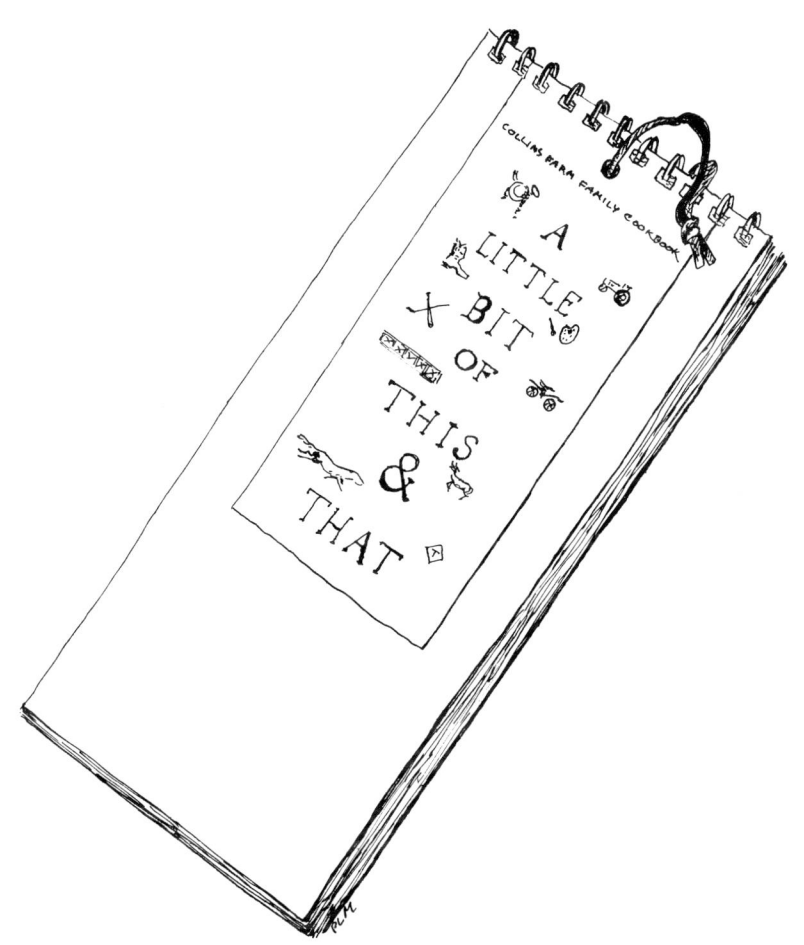

COLLINS FARM FAMILY COOKBOOK

A
LITTLE
BIT
OF
THIS
&
THAT

Guardian Angel
Belva Lee Brissett

"Belva!! There's a long distance call from your doctor in Washington D.C." I remember well that summer day in June 1978. It was bittersweet and unforgettable. We had just received news of the passing of my children's father. The call was to tell Belva the results of her breast biopsy. It was malignant and surgery was needed immediately. After talking with her husband and two children, Belva had her surgery in Oklahoma City.

As her mother and a survivor of breast cancer, I thanked God I was blessed to be able to take care of my daughter at this time. Belva had so unselfishly cared for me during the time of my surgery. It was also consoling to see how supportive Belva's sisters and brothers were during her illness. She could often be heard repeating her motto: "God is able." She was an inspiration.

The women in our family have been haunted by breast cancer for five generations. When Belva recovered, her activism on breast cancer awareness for Black women sparked members of our family to become spokespersons for the American Cancer Society and Breast Cancer Resource Committee (which includes Cancer Awareness Services). Today all my girls and granddaughters know how to check their breasts and take care of themselves.

In the years following her surgery, the bond between my children grew and they shared many happy and sad times. Belva died in 1990. Our family believes God honored Belva's last request to assign her as the guardian angel over the Brown family.

Belva Lee Brissett, of Oklahoma City, died at age 49. Submitted in her memory by her mother, Helen Brown. Belva had been diagnosed initially at age 37. She was a lobbyist for the National Association of Broadcasters in Washington, D.C., later promoted to Senior Vice President. Belva's mother, Helen, is a breast cancer survivor and wishes to dedicate this story in honor of her daughter's life.

The line art on this page, called "Guardian Angel," was drawn by Deborah J. McKinley. Please note other pieces of art which she has created and initialed (DJM) in this book. D.J. was diagnosed with Stage III breast cancer at age 42 in March 1992. She underwent six months of aggressive chemotherapy and 32 rounds of radiation. She is now enjoying life to the fullest and hopes to complete her Master's degree in Art Therapy and "to give back to the Lord something of the precious gift He has given me." She credits her positive attitude to her role model, her 91-year-old grandmother, Virgie Lee Johnston, and says, "Without her inspiration and positive attitude, I would not be where I am today."

Will My Daughter?
Marti Miller

There is a feeling of being sheltered when we look at pictures of loved ones and ancestors. Their strength becomes ours somehow. As we watched breast cancer take the life from our grandmother, Nannie, we knew she only wanted to see her first great-grandchild. Our mother, Marti, cherished the memories of her mother's long, fulfilling life and went on with her own. None of us could imagine the impact breast cancer would have on our family, and how much we would need Nannie's strength.

Four years later, in 1976 at age 53, Mother's worst fear became reality. She entered the hospital, signed very frightening consent forms, and woke up the next day with no breast and extreme pain. She continued with her very active life and sheltered us from the hardest parts. Deep in her heart and ours, we sometimes dared to let the question take form, "Will I have to face breast cancer, too?"

The news remained good for 17 years. Then, in 1992, at age 44, it was my turn. My mother's courage and resolve helped me to have the inner strength to survive as well. It was as if I had been "prepared." But no one was prepared for what happened next. In July 1993, a routine mammogram revealed a suspicious lump in Mother's remaining breast. We regathered our determination to continue our journey together. She is always willing to help someone else "carry the baggage" that must be taken on the same journey.

Our family is now involved with the nationwide familial study. We hope that something about our genetic makeup will give clues to unravel the mysteries of this disease. Yes, we often ponder the question, "Will my daughter or sister have to go on a similar journey?"

Marti Miller, age 72, of Oklahoma City. Submitted by her daughters, Vicki Miller Medlin and Jacki Miller Rhea. Vicki was diagnosed in 1992 and wrote this story. Marti was diagnosed the first time at age 53, and again at age 70. She has been a loving daughter, supportive wife, devoted mother, proud grandmother, and cherished friend. Her daughters describe Marti's life as one that continues to be an inspiration to many.

3
Grit and Determination
"I will survive!"

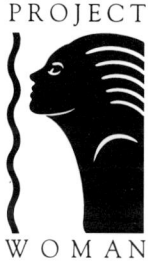

3
Grit and Determination
"I will survive!"

~⌒

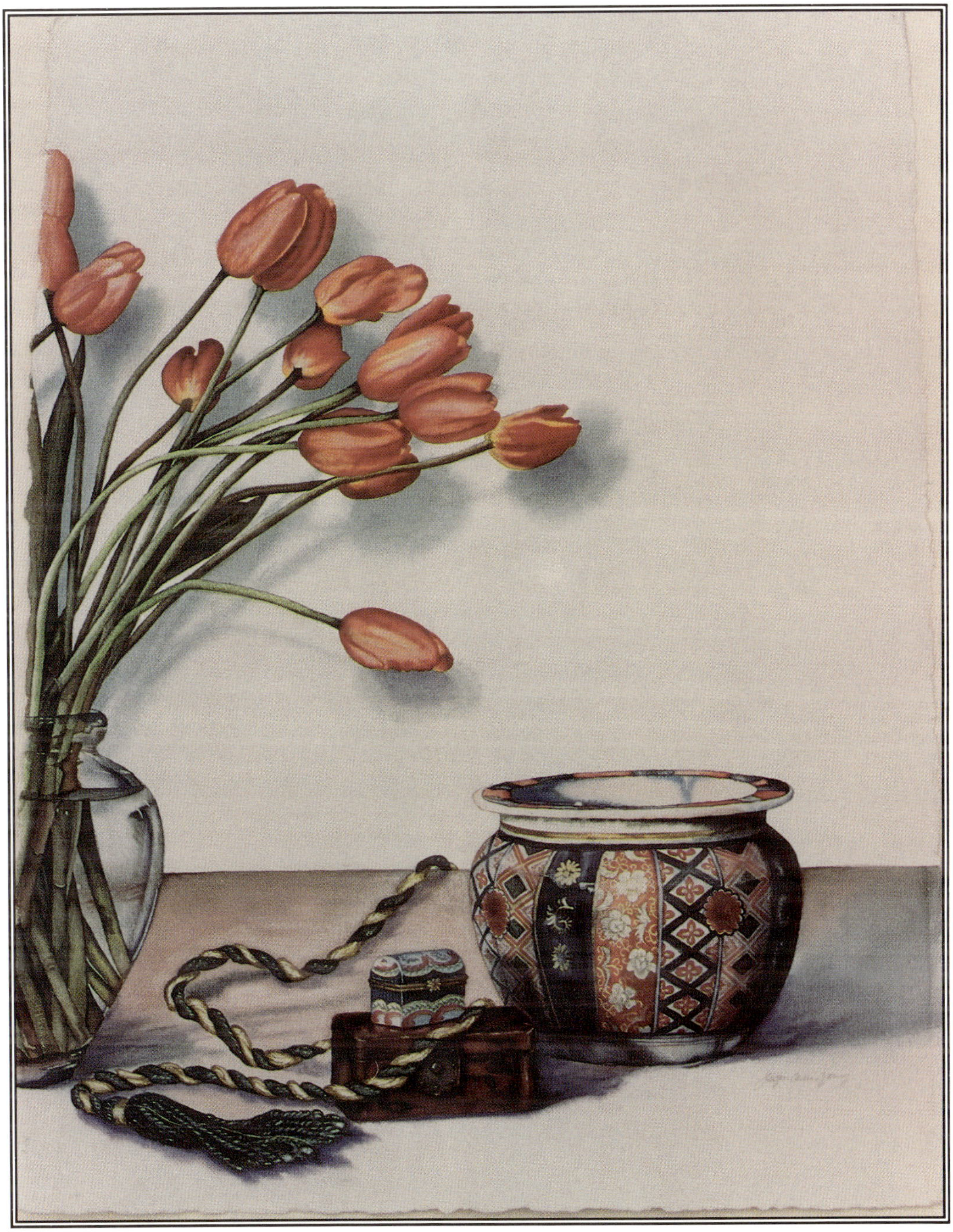

"Tulip Plié"   Jacque Collins Young

I Will Survive

Tammy Mass

I had just graduated from college in the summer of 1983. Less than two months later, I was diagnosed with breast cancer and had a double mastectomy. Just when I thought my life was coming together, it seemed it was falling apart. I had an eight-month old baby, a husband, a college degree and career opportunities to pursue. My world was at stake.

Quickly I came to terms with the inevitable; when push came to shove, my ultimate goal was to live, survive, and recover. I have done all that with the support of my family and friends and a strong belief deep inside me that I'm not going to die. I'm not ready to give up and nothing, but nothing will keep me down. As the song goes, "I will survive."

Each year of survival I feel blessed to receive a clean bill of health. Each year on my cancer anniversary date, I am more optimistic that I have beaten the odds and that I will live to see my two children graduate, go on dates, marry, and have children of their own.

I believe that life's too short to sweat the small stuff. I don't worry as much as I used to about everything being perfect, or fretting over laundry or chores or staying up late, driving a little too fast or turning the radio up loud, speaking my mind when I see injustice, and being honest about my feelings. I maintain a positive attitude and project an optimistic spirit in everything I do as wife, mother, employee.

Tammy Mass, age 35, of Yukon. Tammy was diagnosed at the very early age of 23, and has tried to maintain a positive attitude and project an optimistic spirit in everything she does. Her life is very full. She works full time with Fleming Companies and as an Avon representative. She and her husband have two active children, one in gymnastics and the other in advanced academics. She has great hope for the future and plans to live life to the fullest.

Get Up, Dust Off, Keep Going
Betty Rae Marshall

When I first learned that I had breast cancer, I thought my life was surely over, especially when I considered the prospect of having a mastectomy and six months of intensive chemotherapy. After the initial shock wore off, I decided that I could spend the rest of my life wondering why this had happened to me, or I could do everything possible to make the most of my life. My mother and father were very supportive during my bout with cancer. No one knew they both had cancer at that time also. My mother died in 1989 and, in less than four months, my father died. I hope I helped make a difference for them and made things just a little easier. I had some down times, but my faith in God and my family, friends, and students always helped me to get up, dust off, and keep going.

Betty Rae Marshall, age 46, of Hominy. Betty, a high school English, French, and journalism teacher for 24 years, was diagnosed at age 39. Her husband, Tandy, describes Betty as a happy person who is a positive role model for everyone who knows her. She plays the organ for her church and is president of the women's ministry organization. She is also director of a junior club, a teen club, and a family camp for Modern Woodsmen of America, all family-based organizations which are community oriented.

Same Person I Was
Jane Culwell

I had gone to bed and was lying on my side; my right breast was hurting a little bit and I rubbed my hand across it. Then I felt a lump about the size of a large marble. Within three days I had a mammogram in Dallas. My doctor said we'd better get me to the hospital and check it out. The next day they removed my breast. The doctor told me to call it what it was and not avoid the word cancer. I had six weeks of radiation treatment. I was 39 then. Today, I have been free of cancer for 17 years. I went on with my life and did not let the fact that I lost a breast bother me. I am the same person that I was before. No doubt, the early detection and diagnosis have given me the opportunity to see my children grow up and to enjoy my grandchildren.

Jane Culwell, age 56, of Marietta. Jane, who worked as a secretary/bookkeeper and auto parts clerk, was diagnosed at age 39. She now owns her own garage and machine shop, and is a former member of the Marietta City Council. She is a member of the First Methodist Church.

I Fooled Them
Martha Owens

After the surgery I started chemotherapy. I would leave from school every day at 3:00 to take the treatments. I didn't miss work. If my students asked, I talked about it openly. I did have one student whose mother recently had passed away with cancer, and she was upset. I assured her that I was okay; we became good friends. I thought if I talked to them, it would help them better to understand, if and when someone they knew also became sick. Education about cancer is the best weapon.

The main problem I had was getting tired. All my children and grandchildren came for Christmas that year. They made such a big fuss and took lots of pictures. It was like they thought it was my last Christmas. I fooled them! I've had three more. They don't all come anymore; I think they've discovered I'm going to live.

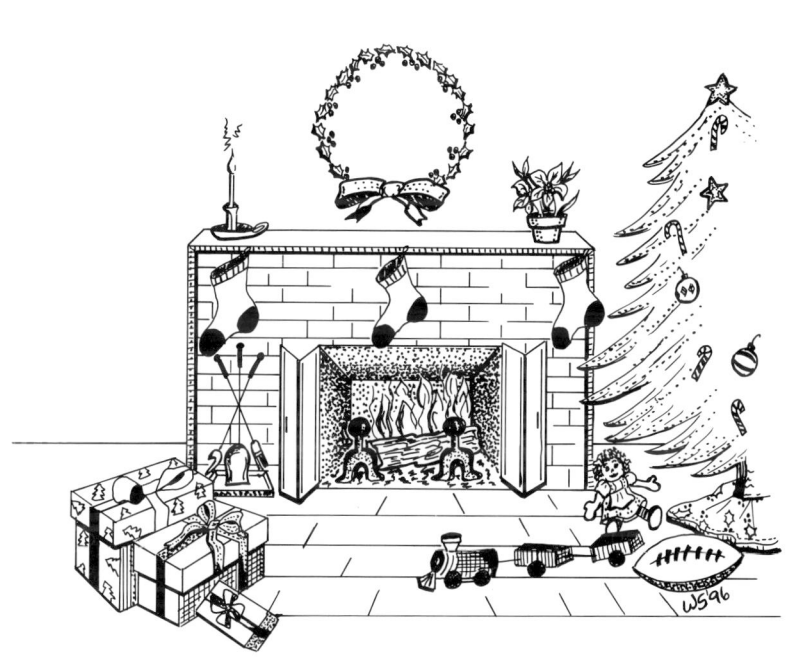

Martha Owens, age 60, of Muskogee. Martha, a teacher of mathematics at Hilldale High School, was diagnosed at age 56. Martha raised four children, then adopted three more. She has ten grandchildren and five great-grandchildren. After becoming a single mother in 1973, she completed college and began her career as a high school math teacher. She has been active in various educational and tennis organizations, as well as a member of the Muskogee Cancer Support Group.

Will to Live
Wilma Sprouse

꘏

I have experienced all the effects in learning I had cancer—the fear, anger, grief, joy, and healing that go with such a diagnosis. But through it all, thank God, I had a sincere desire to live and I had the support of my husband, son, family, friends, and church.

꘏

Wilma Sprouse, age 57, of Henryetta. Wilma works for her church, is active as a community volunteer, and helps others cope with cancer, especially those who are terminally ill. She was initially diagnosed at age 53.

Ups and Downs
Margaret Shipley

꘏

After having had cervical cancer in 1961, Margaret was diagnosed with breast cancer in 1988 at age 72. Despite her ups and downs she keeps going and is uplifting for everyone around her. She has been a breast cancer survivor for eight years now, and is doing great for her age.

꘏

Margaret Shipley, age 79, of Muskogee. Submitted by her friend, Rachel Collins. Margaret was diagnosed at age 72, and had worked in a medical records department in Beaumont, Texas. She later worked as an office manager at a laundry for 30 years and managed apartments following that, where she continues to help the needy who may live there.

Live to the Fullest
Gerri Beeson

꘏

Since my cancer was found very early by a routine mammogram, I did not have to have chemotherapy or radiation. I have done well. Each medical check-up is symptom free. I am living proof that early detection and treatment can take care of the problem and you can get on with your life. I'm planning to retire next year and travel with a backpack through Europe and Russia by rail, bus and boat. I will pass this way but once and I hope to live life to the fullest. Remember what Norman Cousins said: "Whatever is necessary is possible."

꘏

Gerri Beeson, age 61, of Oklahoma City. A teacher and volunteer administrator, Gerri coordinated the volunteer program at the Oklahoma Library for the Blind. She is a member of the Governor's Task Force on Volunteerism, and was a U.S. Peace Corps Volunteer in Africa from 1979–81. Her initial diagnosis was at age 57.

Stubborn and Bull-Headed
Johnnie McWhirter

I went in on Friday to review my records with the surgeon. He read my mammogram and said he didn't like the way my right breast looked, and this was the side I had not even been concerned about. So, on the following Monday, April 4, 1993, I went in for biopsies and awoke with both breasts gone and nearly all my lymph glands removed. Six weeks before the surgery my oldest son and daughter-in-law gave birth to my grandson. I was a very crazy Nana and adored Dalton. I was going to fight for my life. People have told me that I am stubborn and bull-headed, but this is what it has taken to survive.

We traveled to M.D. Anderson Hospital in Houston to get a second opinion on the method of treatment I should receive. They were not very encouraging at all. I returned home and began eight weeks of aggressive chemotherapy treatments at a closer location so my friends and family could be there for support.

In September 1993, I began a bone marrow transplant. During this time I had no immune system and something as simple as a cold would have been deadly for me. My grandson would be brought to my window for me to see and I watched him on home videos. In March 1994, I was diagnosed with acute pancreatitis. After several unsuccessful attempts to return to my teaching job, that I so dearly love, I was forced to ask for disability retirement. The pancreatitis attacks continued to occur.

I have a close friend who was also taking chemo treatments after his sixth round with cancer. This year he and I will both be 50 years old. We always said that we will not mourn over being a half century old, but rejoice if we make it there because we consider ourselves a miracle.

Although my upper body has many scars and is very swollen and tender, I am able to live a happy life and continue to enjoy the small things in life so many people take for granted. My grandchildren give me lots of hugs, kisses and love, and I am able to give them love in return. Only because of my faith in God and the many prayers from people all over the world, am I alive today.

Johnnie McWhirter, age 50, of Maysville. An elementary school teacher, day care operator and teacher, farmer's wife, mother and grandmother, Johnnie was diagnosed at age 47. She is a member of several education associations, the FFA Mother's Club, the Oklahoma Farm Bureau, and the Lindsay Activity Booster Club.

Coming to Terms with the Thing I Fear Most
Karen Pewthers-Yirak

'Tis not Death—
That mighty fearful dread
That scares us all,
Though some doth come to terms before the end.
No.
'Tis something quieter.
More silent than hot summer stillness,
More hidden than shadows at night,
Something unspoken… turned away from… not allowed.
My breasts are gone.
And thee with thine own two soft masses of flesh
Doth go on without thinking, without understanding my loss.
Just replace them, ye sayeth,
Get fixed.
Wear falsies.
Things will be just like they were.
Nay.
I think not.
I lost more than my breasts that year.
I lost my social sexuality.
I lost my leverage as well as my cleavage.
I lost part of my tools.
And that, then, is what I fear most.
Can I make it, without being defined by this body?
… Or in spite of it?
Will thine and thee look past my straight form to value the ME?
Who is still quite sexual, by the way…
And beyond that, will I be able to move past the misplaced, awkward shame
To a self-embrace of serene acceptance, where I would redefine my self image and feel
Content? Secure?
That, then, will be coming to terms with the thing I fear most.
That, then, will be my healing.

Karen Pewthers-Yirak, age 48, of Oklahoma City. Karen describes herself as an "experimenter in creativity, experiencer of fun and life, and seeker of truth and light." She was diagnosed at age 44.

I Have More to Do
Pat Bowles

❧

I have a positive attitude about living with cancer which I hope will encourage other patients, survivors, and their families. Life goes on. I was back teaching exercise classes three months after my mastectomy and I taught while taking chemotherapy. My friends say I have "energy plus." The word cancer did not scare me. I'm too determined to live. I have more to do.

❧

Pat Bowles, age 57, of Duncan. Pat, diagnosed at age 47, is a mother, homemaker, and volunteer. She discovered aerobic dancing at age 39, which led her to a career as an aerobics instructor in Duncan for 12 years. After treatment for breast cancer, Pat is proud to say she is back teaching senior adult exercise classes.

Embraced by an Angel
Wanda Higgins

❧

Wanda: "We can't control the things that happen to us, but we can control our attitude."

Teresa: "Mother loves to give hugs and they are the best! When she hugs me I feel like I've been embraced by an angel."

❧

Wanda Higgins, age 55, of Yukon. Submitted by her daughter, Teresa Buhl. Wanda, who was diagnosed at age 54, was a medical assistant and office manager for a surgeon, followed by a position as a computer operator for a local CPA firm. She is a devoted wife, mother, and grandmother, active in church and her grandchildren's sports and school activities.

When I Am Gone
Jerry Ann Elmenhorst

❧

When I am gone it is only goodbye for a short time. I want to spend eternity with all of you. Won't that be a wonderful celebration!

❧

Jerry Ann Elmenhorst, of El Reno, died at age 54. Submitted in her memory by her daughter, Cindy Sharum. Jerry was first diagnosed at age 39; the second diagnosis came at age 51. A wife and mother of five, she was a grandmother of nine. She became a licensed practical nurse in 1987. Her second diagnosis came while she was in school studying to become an LPN. Her daughter, Cindy, feels her mother was and can still be an example to other women with breast cancer because she never gave up.

I Want to Live, and That's What Counts
Mary Battenfield

It happened to me on a Sunday evening at bedtime. I was removing my T-shirt when I felt a tender spot in my left breast. My heart jumped to my throat. I called to my physician husband to come feel this "thing." We reassured each other that although it was a lump, it was probably benign. After all, cancer didn't run in my family so it would be okay. But the nagging question, "What if it isn't benign?" led me finally to make an appointment with the Ob/Gyn, who promptly sent me to the radiologist for a mammogram. No one said too much, but they did point out areas of concern. I don't know if it was the blood rushing so hard in my ears or my heart beating so loud, but I did not comprehend that there were more than two lumps.

I was in the hospital talking with the surgeon the night before the surgery when the full impact of what was happening hit me. He asked me what I wanted him to do if it was cancer. I replied, "Do what you would do for your wife!" I went into surgery fairly certain the lumps were cancerous. Sure enough, when I awakened with the left side of my body hurting, I knew. But I was not going to let this get me down. I transferred my body from the gurney to the bed almost completely on my own power. We had things to do—so naturally, I would have to get well quickly.

It was decided that I would receive chemotherapy then radiation, the treatments of choice for my particular cancer. Before my first treatment, I was warned that I would need a wig because the Cytoxan usually makes one lose her hair. I went to a men's hairpiece shop and ordered a synthetic wig. I had my first treatment. It was ba-a-a-d!! I accused the oncologist of trying to kill me. He said, "Yes, but just a little short of it." Not funny! Before two weeks had gone by, I was driving down the street with my window rolled down and my hair began to blow out the window. I had to laugh and tell this story just to prove I could talk about it. I hated losing my hair and I hated losing my breast, but I was alive and that's what counted.

I went through all the chemotherapy treatments bravely but hating and dreading every minute of it. One tries not to complain, but it makes you so sick. I threw up so much and spent so much time in my bathroom, I decided then and there I would change that wallpaper I hated so much when I got better. I never wanted to look at myself in the mirror without my hair; feeling the shaved head was bad enough, so I always wore my wig or a turban. When I see pictures of me back then, I wince at the sunken, dark-rimmed eyes. I recall the smell of the chemicals and the dread. That was the loneliest time because no one could do it for me. But I reminded myself—I'm alive and that's what counts.

What I really longed for was someone with whom I could talk and commiserate on my own terms and who had been through what I had been through. I didn't know of anyone who had exactly the same set of problems I did. I knew of no support groups to join. My family and friends were my support group. And what a support group they were and still are. They were my cheerleaders and mood lifters. I am so grateful to be alive, and that's what matters to me.

After chemotherapy ended, we went on a trip to Colorado to view the fall foliage before I was to begin radiation treatment. They pinpointed my skin and made me my very own mold for the radiation. This treatment was to be easier and harder in some ways. I was not nauseated, but towards the end of the daily treatments, my skin began to burn, which was of course the object—to sear those bad cells.

Christmas was coming and I felt like a zombie. I forced myself to get ready and do all the traditional things you do at Christmas. After Christmas, one busy day followed another. I had to keep busy, otherwise I would dwell on myself. I'm the "eternal enabler" in the family. But I realized I needed to do something for myself, something exciting; so I went into business with a friend. I worked so hard I couldn't think about a recurrence. Occasionally, I would think I was getting cancer again because my breast would feel tender. My mind would play tricks on me. I would have forgotten that I had on the previous day sawed limbs off a tree or done some other strenuous activity. I was going to be fine. I had to be. I wanted to live and that's what counted.

I really anticipated my five-year anniversary milestone because I knew that meant I was doing great. Wrong! It was explained to me that with the nodal involvement I had, probably a ten-year anniversary celebration would be more appropriate. I remember saying to the doctor one day, "Well, just how bad was it?" He replied, "With 19 of 38 nodes positive, it was certainly not good." I was stunned. Still, I knew I was going to be fine. I had to be. I wanted to live.

I kept busy. I knew other women that had been diagnosed after me and they had succumbed to breast cancer. I did not dare find out their particulars; it might be just the same as mine. My tenth anniversary rolled around. My husband pointed out that I had the same life expectancy as his now, if not better. And, he added offhandedly, that with a 25% chance of living, I had certainly beaten the odds. What? Was I nuts? Did I hear him right? Why didn't I know that? Did I know that? Did it just slip by me? Would I have given up with such poor odds? I honestly don't know.

I do not take the simple joys of life for granted. I love the birds, people, working in the yard, travelling, playing with the grandchildren. I'm going to be fine. I have to be. I want to live, and that's what counts!

Mary Battenfield, age 57, of Tulsa. Mary was an elementary school teacher for eight years. She spent many years raising a family and trying to make the world a better place, whether it was by planting a tree in the school yard or giving away everything in her suitcase while in Africa. Diagnosed at age 45, Mary is an unofficial goodwill ambassador for Oklahoma, and has travelled to 66 countries, including China and Russia.

My Enemy
Mary Jane McIlvain

I have met you, I have glimpsed your face.
     So far, in only one form.
But I know you have many disguises
     As you slither your way into a human organism.

It seems only fair to warn you however,
     You cannot win, no matter how hard you try.
Come any way you will, use all your tricks and tools,
     Your days are numbered.

We are onto your ways, and in the end
     We will conquer you.
But, if it doesn't come soon,
     I have my own battlefield on which to face you.

And this you need to know beforehand:
     You are outnumbered three to one.
Because you see, I have my heart, my mind, and my spirit,
     And these you cannot down.

No matter how you strike, in the stillness of the night,
     Or openly and blatantly for all to see.
It is also fair to warn you
     I hold a secret weapon you cannot comprehend.

God is on my side and even you must rest, but He is ever present.

Mary Jane McIlvain, age 76, of Woodward. Mary Jane, an elementary school teacher, wife, mother of two and grandmother of six, was diagnosed at the age of 56. She is quite active in her church, is Vice President of the Woodward Educational Foundation, and is a volunteer for Reach to Recovery.

To Live Once More
Donna R. Brown

Divorced, on my own, needing reassurance
and now, God, you cast this deathly burden.

It is love, support of my feelings of abandonment
that I crave but now I have anger.

I will not die, no, not now will I crumble.
This battle is lost but not the war.

And, with "Thy will be done…" I survived
to live once more with love and my own earned reassurance.

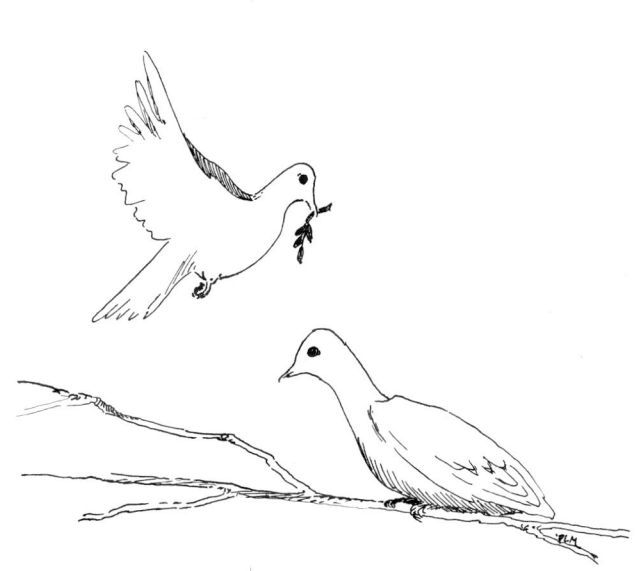

Donna R. Brown, age 59, of Oklahoma City. Donna is the Eldercare case manager for the Logan County County Health Department, and was initially diagnosed at age 55.

The Miracle Child
Teresa Curtis

In June of 1990 I turned 30 years old. In the previous month, my husband had felt a hard place in my right breast. I watched it for several weeks hoping it would go away, but it didn't. It became so painful that I made an appointment with my family physician to have it checked out. When the doctor later told me I had cancer, I was shocked. I called my mother who tried to convince me that most breast lumps are not cancerous and that it would be O.K. She reminded me that her mother had had a radical mastectomy at age 24 and was now in her 80s, and that my aunt had had a modified radical mastectomy ten years earlier and both women had survived; so there was no reason I couldn't be a survivor also. The next week I learned that I had a malignant tumor in my right breast and a benign tumor in the left breast. I just started crying. I was so naive that I had always thought "malignant" meant you would die and "benign" meant you would live. I knew I wasn't ready to die.

Because my cancer was advanced and I was so young, they decided to start me on a high-dose chemotherapy treatment schedule. The biggest fear in my whole life was needles, and here I was being poked every two weeks. I kept joking with the nurses that I should be getting used to needles, but they assured me no one gets used to them. You just tolerate them; you do what you have to do.

One of my greatest physical assets was my hair. I frequently got compliments on it. I had read that not everyone will lose their hair from chemotherapy so I became optimistic that I would not lose mine. But then the oncologist assured me that Adriamycin (also known as "the red devil") would definitely cause hair loss. I first noticed my hair was falling out while taking a shower, shortly after my second chemo treatment. I was shocked, and though I was expecting it, I just started crying. Then later, several members of my church told me their children had no idea I had been wearing a wig. Ah, out of the mouths of babes. They inspired a new attitude in me toward people wearing wigs. It was, at times, even humorous. Once I was putting a carryout pizza in the back seat of my car and my wig attached itself to the roof of my car just like velcro!

Because of the high recurrence rate for my stage of cancer, the doctors thought it best that I not have reconstruction right after my mastectomy. So after waiting 12 months from the time my final treatment was completed, I was given permission to have the TRAM-flap method done. Also because of the risks of recurrence, the doctors highly advised that I wait to try to have a baby. The thinking was that the increased hormonal activity brought on by pregnancy could accelerate the growth of any dormant cells that might not be detected, thereby increasing the risk of recurrence. So we decided to wait until the summer of 1993 to have a baby; but God's time table was different, and on March 30, 1993, we had what my mother calls our "miracle child," Olivia. Fortunately, there have been no signs of any health problems for her. I was able to breast feed her for 14 months with only the left breast. I never had any soreness or cracked nipple, and I always had plenty of milk for her.

A few weeks after I weaned Olivia, I was due for my annual mammogram on the left breast. Afterwards, that Friday afternoon, my family physician called to say they had found a suspicious place that they wanted me to have biopsied. The shock was almost worse than the original diagnosis four years earlier. All I knew was that never again could I face emotionally this kind of scare. I made up my mind to have the left breast removed whether it was cancerous or not. So, in June of 1994 I had a simple mastectomy with a tissue expander inserted. The lump was found to be benign; no lymph nodes were removed and no additional treatment was necessary. I elected to have immediate reconstruction; this time I chose a silicone implant.

After all the surgery and chemo and radiation, I feel confident I made the right decisions and I now have assurance that I will never get breast cancer again. I may still be at risk of a recurrence in another part of my body, but for now I see myself living a long, full life.

Postscript: Teresa Was an Answer to My Prayer
by Gail Jackson
(mother of Teresa Curtis)

I had two sons and my husband said he didn't want any more children after he was 25 years old. I prayed that I would be given a girl. That prayer was answered on June 5, 1960—Teresa was born. Thirty years later, when she told me that it was suspected she had breast cancer, my heart sank. My mother had breast cancer at age 24. My older sister had breast cancer at age 50. There were lots of tears, but I never once thought I would lose Teresa. Later, 14 months after her radiation treatments, we were thrilled to learn that she was pregnant, but I worried about her and the baby's health. I prayed that all would be well. Again, my prayers were answered when Olivia was born on March 30, 1993. Such a pretty child. I called her our "miracle child." By the way, Mother is now 85 years old and still going strong.

Teresa Curtis, age 35, of Edmond. Teresa was initially diagnosed at age 30, and wishes to be an encouragement to those who have breast cancer and to give hope that there is life after breast cancer.

Beat the Odds
Jodi Liese

My doctors told me, after the fourth recurrence of my disease: "You will have to make your own statistics because you have outlived most of ours."

I hope that will encourage others to fight on so we can make long term prognoses for many!

Jodi Liese, age 47, of Guymon. Jodi, a mother, homemaker, substitute teacher and foster parent, was diagnosed at age 36. She is active as a Girl Scout leader, Cub Scout leader, and church volunteer as well as a foster parent for 94 children from 1972 to 1994. Her prayer is to live long enough to raise her children.

There's Always Someone Less Fortunate
Yvonne Jim

I have had the unfortunate experience of getting breast cancer not only once in my life but twice. I was 28 years old when I was first diagnosed; then again 12 years later. I told my nurse that I was just happy to be alive and losing a breast was not going to keep me from living on. I look around me at work, on the street, read the paper, and say to myself, "There is always someone less fortunate than I." Besides I know the Lord has plans for me because during my latest diagnosis, I was told I will be having my third child.

Yvonne Jim, age 40, of Wewoka. Yvonne was diagnosed the first time at age 28 and the second time at age 40. She is a purchasing agent with the Indian Health Service where she has been employed since 1977. With her second diagnosis came an unexpected blessing—she became pregnant with her third child. She has been married for 21 years and knows she has and always will have a lot of love and support from her family.

Surviving
Margaret Louise Long

In August, 1988, Joe, Meg, Jim, my husband, and I planned a getaway to Boston, Massachusetts. A few days before we were scheduled to go, Meg found a small lump in her left breast while doing a routine breast examination. She quickly made an appointment to have it checked. It was decided to biopsy the lump. Everyone was positive it would be benign. Meg was told she might be a bit sore, but to go on to Boston and have a good time. But, it was malignant. The doctor performed a modified radical mastectomy which, it was decided, would require no further treatment.

We were all elated. The philosophy we had was to approach all situations head on, with an amazingly positive attitude, a joke, and a laugh or two, and the resolve to get through and move on to greener pastures. And so we did.

Then Joe was offered the opportunity to teach at the University of Louisville Law School during the Fall 1989 semester. He accepted. In August, Meg and Joe went to Louisville, set up house for Joe, and Meg flew back. She was scheduled for her annual checkup the day after returning from Louisville. Want to guess what was found? You got it—three small lumps, barely detectable by the doctor. We called Joe and he returned to Norman. Meg underwent surgery to remove the lumps, followed by intensive chemotherapy/radiation treatments. I thought she would never survive.

But, remember our general philosophy? Of course, it was not as simple as a smile and a happy attitude. Like the following November, for example, we decided to reschedule the trip to Boston, Mass. Second verse? Same as the first. Meg went to the hospital with pneumonia. It was a tough, miserable time for Meg and Joe. None of us thought she would be around for the holidays.

Fortunately, for a multitude of family and friends, Meg did survive. She fought the demon and won. At the age of 50, Meg became the longest surviving female in her direct family line.

The moral of this story: DO NOT ever plan a trip to Boston, Massachusetts with the Longs or Ringos. Life is too precious and we're jinxed!

Margaret "Meg" Long, age 51, of Norman. Submitted by her friend, Robin Ringo. Meg was diagnosed at age 44, while serving as a homemaker and volunteer. She is on the board of the American Cancer Society's Cleveland County Unit, and chair of Operation School Bell, a project which clothes over 700 children each year. A wife and mother of two, Meg is very determined to beat cancer and to see her boys through school.

Fifteen Years and Holding
Clara Wichert

It was June 1979. We were in wheat harvest. I had just left the wheat truck to go in for a cold shower. What a surprise to feel a lump in my left breast. Quickly I searched the opposite breast. Yes! There it was, same size and position. Adrenalin rushed through my body and fear filled my soul. What would my future bring?

A mammogram was finally ordered. Report: No need for surgery. Just "watch" the lumps for changes. We waited. Months passed. We watched. My appetite disappeared. I became extremely tired. In April 1980, on my 40th birthday, a biopsy was performed. Cancer in both breasts.

The "C" word was not publicly discussed back then. I had no one to talk to. My parents waited for me to die. The only people they knew who had cancer, died. My husband and two sons were in shock.

I survived two separate surgeries, one week apart, breast tissue, all muscle and lymph nodes and two large skin grafts from each upper thigh to cover the exposed area. But a miracle was in the making. Wow! I arrived home after four weeks. The following evening I was escorted down the aisle by my son Rex (16), three tubes, bandages, and all, and watched as my older son, Jeff, took his marriage vows.

Well, two years of chemo (the old fashioned way) certainly caused me to think that death might have been easier. But today, 15 years later, I feel like the richest lady in town. I have health (Thanks, Lord); wealth (many friends); and the love of a good man! (I love you, Loyd). My prayer is: "Lord, each day you give me, help me to make a difference!"

Clara Wichert, age 55, of Fairview. Clara, a homemaker, was diagnosed at age 40. She has been extremely active in her community, including serving as chair of the Major County Farm Bureau Women's Club, volunteering for Meals on Wheels, the Bloodmobile, Ag in the Classroom, Reach to Recovery, and Children's Director of the Mennonite Brethren Church.

Death's Door
Nancy "Rosy" Glenn

I stood at death's threshold, the door flung open wide,
suspended between Life and Death, waiting to go inside.

I lingered at the threshold, dancing on the brink,
hanging in the balance, not knowing what to think.

Beyond the door a brightness such as I have never seen
and in the midst, Jesus; great peace came over me.

The suffering cannot compare to the end of life's race;
vanished all my fears with one look upon his face.

He knew the anguish;
He knew the pain.

He had conquered this very threshold
that eternity I might gain.

O' Death where is thy sting?
Grave, where is thy victory?

Just beyond death's door,
Rejoicing evermore!

Nancy "Rosy" Glenn, age 39, of Tulsa. Rosy is a dedicated wife, mother, homemaker, and professional in the health care field. She does public health promotions for the Women/Infants/Children program for Tulsa City-Tulsa County Health Department, serves as a Sunday school teacher, and teaches nutrition education to low income families. Rosy was 37 when she was diagnosed.

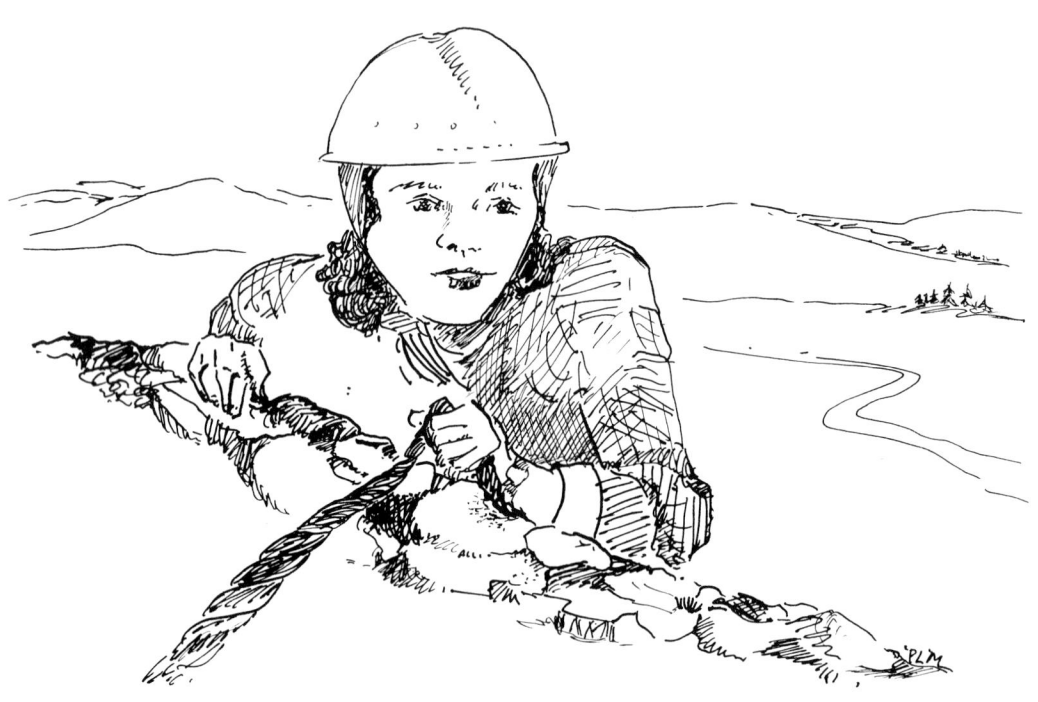

I'll Climb My Mountain
Sharon Weeks

When I first heard that the needle biopsy showed cancer, I was numb. I was gripped with fear that my life would soon be over. I was physically and emotionally ill. I couldn't sit still. I lost my appetite for food. My stomach felt nervous and my intestines constantly felt like snakes or wiggly worms.

I wasn't ready to die. I didn't want to leave my husband or daughters or sons-in-law or grandchildren or friends. I wanted to see my daughter's unborn baby. I wanted to enjoy my grandchildren. I wanted to finish the afghan I had been working on for so long.

Then I prayed, "God, if you want me now, I'm ready. I won't argue or complain, but if you don't, please let me know so I can fight this disease with all I've got." I believe He answered my prayer through my daughter, Shelly. She said, "Mom, we're going to fight this!" I knew then a battle was ahead of me but I also knew I had the support of many people and most importantly, God.

Through chemo and radiation treatments and even to this time, I have feelings of fear, pain, depression, frustration, and hope. These feelings come and go and come again. I learned very quickly that I was no longer in control of many facets of my life. Each morning when I awaken, one of my first thoughts is, "I have cancer. This isn't just a terrible dream, it is real." I can no longer do some of the things I loved to do, such as teach, play ball with grandchildren, go on long bicycle rides, play tennis, snow ski, or climb mountains. My mountain is Cancer.

I'm trying to be more patient, to take one day at a time and enjoy each moment. I don't know what discomforts await me, but with God's love, mercy, and ever-presence, and the support of my loved ones, I'll climb my mountain and I'll reach the top.

Sharon Weeks, age 55, of Oklahoma City. Sharon taught fourth grade in public schools for 21 years. She is also a wife, mother and grandmother. She was originally diagnosed with inflammatory breast cancer at age 50 and experienced metastasis to the bone at 52.

4
Laughing through the Tears
"We have to laugh, or we'll cry."

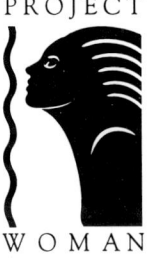

PROJECT

WOMAN

4
Laughing through the Tears
"We have to laugh, or we'll cry."

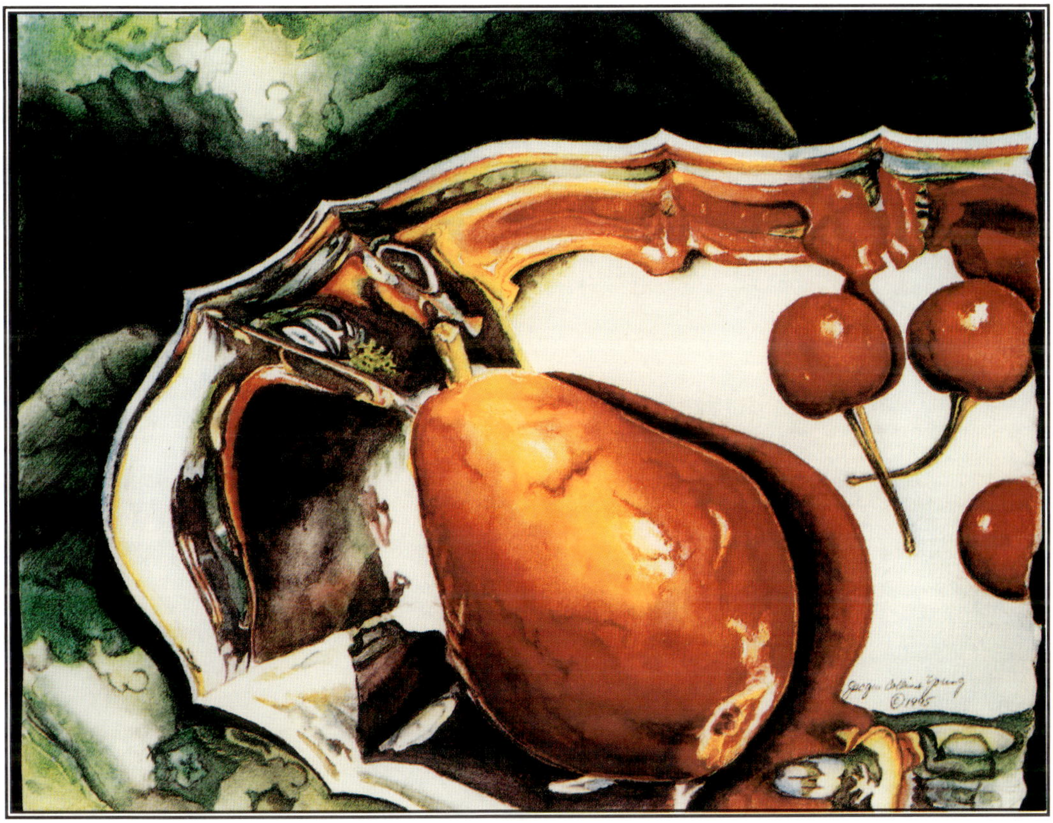

"Scarlet Echoes"   Jacque Collins Young

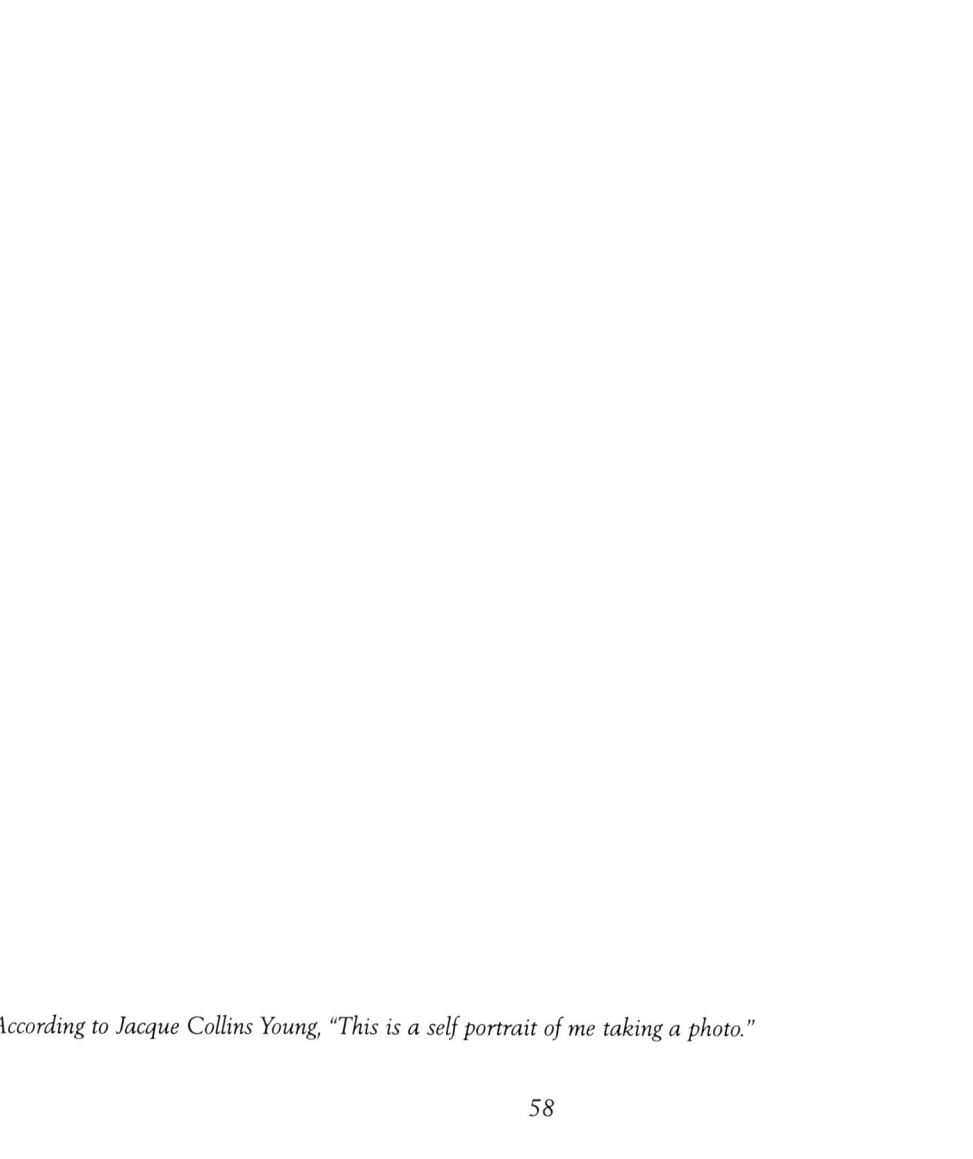

According to Jacque Collins Young, "This is a self portrait of me taking a photo."

Laughing through the Tears
Phala Crownover

I went to the doctor with abdominal pains. He immediately set me up for a battery of tests including a mammogram. I tried to talk him out of it. It was my stomach, not my breasts, that was giving me problems. Fortunately, he didn't listen to me. The next morning when my doctor walked into the examining room, he was not smiling. I began to feel very uneasy. Then came the bombshell! There was a tumor in my left breast, and he was sure it was malignant.

What a shock! How could this be? I had felt nothing during my regular self-examinations. He said it could not be felt because it was at the rear of the breast. Fear suddenly hit me. My mother, sister and several other female relatives had had breast cancer. They were all deceased.

Three weeks later, I saw the surgeon. I could now feel the tumor through my clothes. It had tripled in size. I had a modified radical mastectomy that afternoon. I had made up my mind before I went in for the surgery, that I was going to win this battle. Now, eight years later and with the total support of a loving husband and family, I know I have won!

I am so lucky to be alive. If it were not for the mammogram, I probably wouldn't be. One of the things that has helped me to survive is a sense of humor. Laughing through the tears, anger and fear—I never gave in to negative feelings.

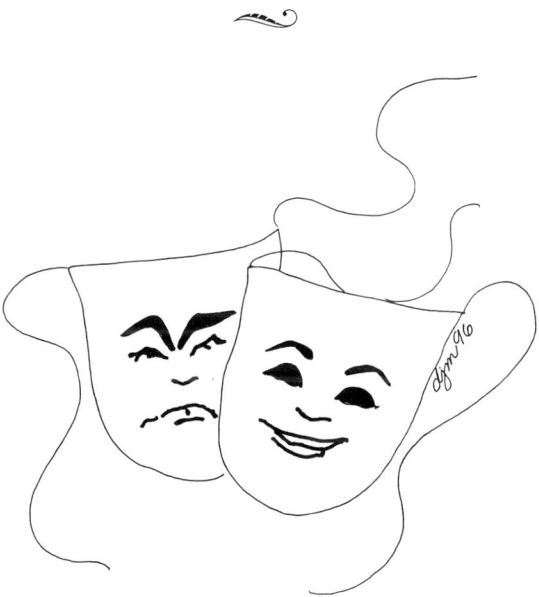

Phala Crownover, age 67, of El Reno. A musician performing since she was five years old, Phala was diagnosed at age 59. She has been a church organist for 50 years, and started acting in 1979. She continues to improve at her arts, and wants to act professionally.

We Have to Laugh, or We'll Cry
Pat Lynn Moses

In 1988, my mother died of multiple myeloma, cancer of the bone marrow. In 1989, my husband's mother, who had survived many years after breast cancer with metastasis to the bone, succumbed to heart disease. In February 1990, I encountered breast cancer myself. I had a lumpectomy, followed a few days later by surgery to install a "port." Most often lumpectomies are performed when only one lump is present and it is no more than two centimeters in size. The pathologist's report showed three tumors, with one over three centimeters, and cancerous cells in over one-third of the lymph nodes removed. My oncologists (I consulted two) decided I should have six months of aggressive chemotherapy followed by six weeks of radiation therapy.

About two weeks after my surgeries, my husband Dale lost his job suddenly. We were given less than a month to move out of the apartment we had occupied as part of his employment. I melted into nausea and fatigue from the chemo; Dale was immobilized with worry and depression. If charted on one of those "Stress Scales," we were definitely way over the top!

Our children and friends packed our belongings and helped move Dale back to our home in Oklahoma City. I headed for Vermont to complete the Master's Degree in art therapy which I'd begun a year before, and to finish my chemotherapy with another oncologist. Dale searched for a new career while I launched into very intensive classwork and the last half of chemotherapy—miles away from the physical support of each others' arms. You can imagine our phone bills! Early on we decided to use every means at our disposal to hold ourselves together, and humor was right up there with eating carrots and taking naps. Often we said, "We have to laugh, or we'll cry!" Of course we cried too, and sometimes we laughed until we cried.

I lost all my hair, but people came up to me and said, "You have the prettiest shaped head." I have always loved hats and scarves, and scarves draped and knotted dramatically look much better on a bald head than over hair. At the end of the summer, my classmates decided to have a big party to celebrate our survival, and chose to have a "Hat Party." Everyone wore elaborately decorated hats, and a prize was to be given for the best hat. I, of course, had been wearing hats, caps, scarves and all sorts of head coverings all summer, except when I chose to go "au naturel." I decided to use a therapeutic art approach and painted my head! I won the prize. The prize turned out to be a bottle of wine, which I could not drink because of my chemotherapy; the "losers" shared it all around.

When I returned home, I began radiation therapy. Every day, week after week, I exposed myself to that lovely machine in the company of compassionate professionals. Just as I approached the end of it, they tacked on a few more weeks for extra precaution. Finally, I arrived for my last treatment—truly a cause for celebration. So, I painted my chest. Huge flowers, trailing vines and leaves in bright strokes of color greeted those staid professionals when I bared myself to the machine that day. My radiation oncologist said, "I've been doing this for 14 years, and I thought I'd seen everything, but I have never seen anything like this!"

It's been six years now, and I remain closely under my physician's care. I try to eat right and exercise regularly, do relaxation and visualization exercises, participate in support programs, make time for emotional and spiritual growth, and appreciate the wonderful support of my family and friends. And, I still count heavily on my sense of humor and my art to keep me going.

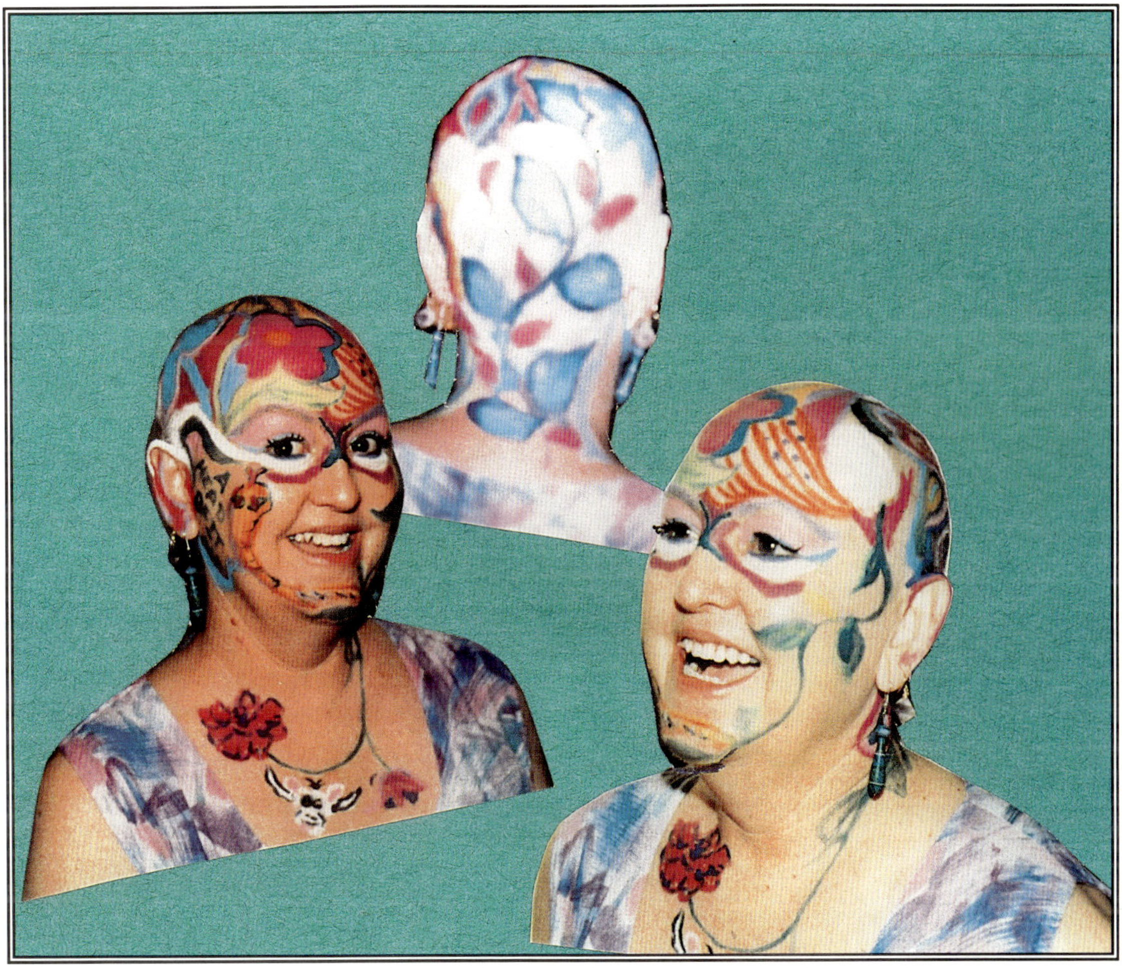

Pat Lynn Moses, age 54, of Oklahoma City. Pat was diagnosed at age 48. She is an art therapist at the Troy & Dollie Smith Cancer Center at INTEGRIS Baptist Medical Center, and works regularly with people diagnosed with cancer, as well as their families.

Precious Moments
Gennie Johnson

After my first chemotherapy treatment, almost all my hair had come out, except for a few scraggly parts. I was looking pretty awful and feeling extremely low. My son, Brent, came home from work. As he was walking toward my bathroom, I yelled to him that I looked terrible. He took one look at me and said, "Mom, you don't look so bad, just flip a wig on," and grinned. I did tie a scarf around my head. Later, when he came down to dinner, he had a bandanna on his head; and my husband, seeing this, came in with one on also. We were a pretty funny looking group!

I became known as E.T. around our house. This was just one of our precious moments during this time.

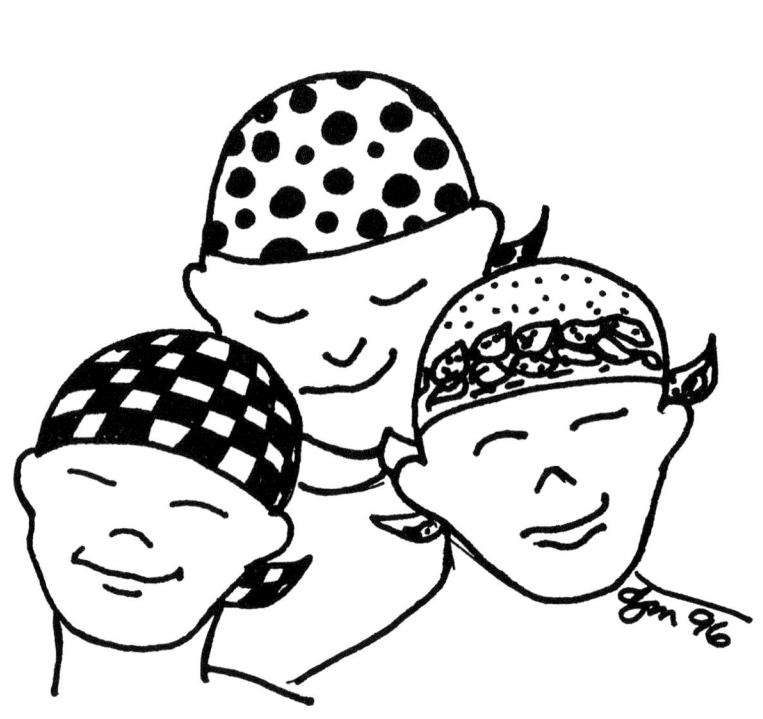

Gennie Johnson, age 53, of Oklahoma City. Gennie, diagnosed at age 48, is an extremely active volunteer in the Oklahoma City community. She has served as Festival of the Arts chair, and on the Festival's executive committee. She is president of the Oklahoma County Bar Auxiliary, in addition to her avid support of cancer-related organizations. She began a breast cancer support group in Oklahoma City called "Bosom Buddies," and was chair of an Oscar de la Renta Fashion Show to raise money for breast cancer awareness.

Lots of Love and Laughter
Tracy A. Turner

Tracy's experience, at age 31, brings home the message that cancer is not a respecter of age. She demonstrates that a beautiful young woman can have breast cancer and still embrace life with zeal. Cancer may have taken a breast from Tracy but it has not taken Tracy. Tracy can bring lightheartedness to the heaviest moments. How many people do you know that can bring the house down making light of being bald and having a portable breast. Tracy can! As she put it, "Survival is all about keeping the human spirit alive while experiencing things that have the potential to crush it. Lots of love and laughter have been a vital part of my recovery. My advice to friends and family of those facing cancer is, 'Just be there.' Your loving presence provides a positive source of energy for the cancer survivor to draw upon when needed."

Tracy Turner, age 31, of Yukon. Submitted by her friends, Pamela Hiti and Susan Lamb. Tracy, an administrative assistant, was diagnosed at age 30. She is an active community volunteer for various health awareness causes including being an AIDS Walk volunteer, a RAIN team leader, a REST volunteer at that group's dental clinic, a teacher of second graders at the Unitarian church school, and a member of Volunteers on Mission, assisting the dentist who organized this program for the United Methodist Church.

It Itches
Terry Gonsoulin

A child's innocence and a sense of humor: two remedies for keeping a positive attitude in spite of breast cancer. What can you do but laugh when…driving home from work, your head is itching so darn bad from the wig, and your four-year-old son reaches over and just yanks the wig right off your bald head and says, "Well, if it itches, Mommy, just take it off!" Of course, the look of shock and horror on the family's faces in the car next to us was worth the laugh the rest of the way home.

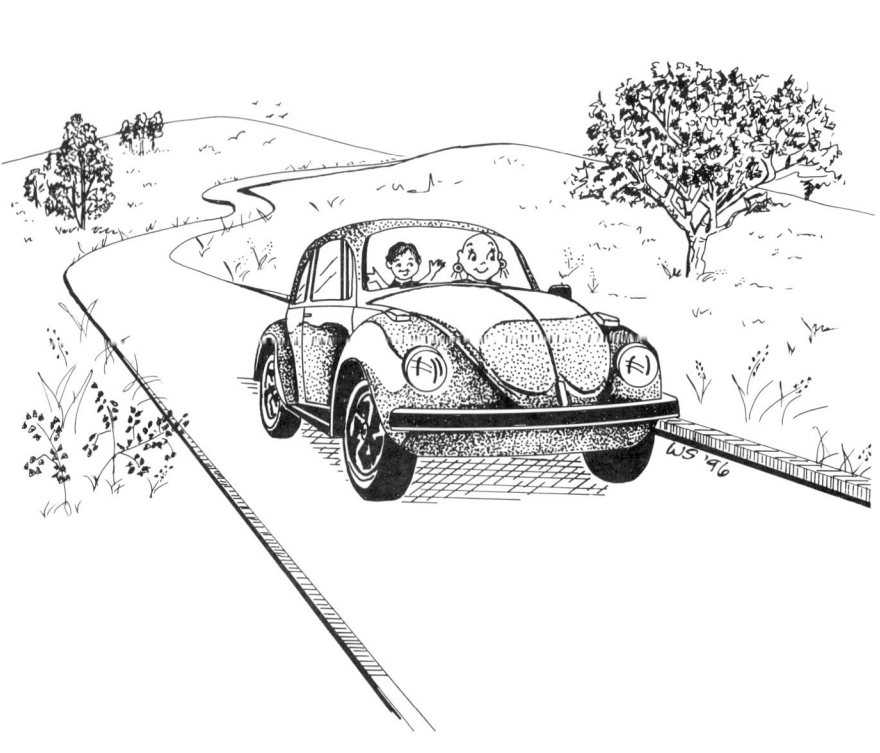

Neighborhood Fashion Show
Terry Gonsoulin

Most people kick their shoes off
when coming home from a hard days work.

I pulled my wig off.

Most women with wigs also carefully
place them on a wig stand.

Mine was hung on the dining chair back.

Until the day I discovered
my wig had disappeared.

It was being passed
from one child's head to another

in the front yard

with the most spectacular imitation
of modeling you have ever seen.

Terry Gonsoulin, age 39, of Oklahoma City. Terry is a registered nurse and serves as administrative director of the Troy & Dollie Smith Cancer Center at INTEGRIS Baptist Medical Center in Oklahoma City. Terry, diagnosed at age 31, is also a wife and mother. She is active in several cancer-related organizations, and is chair of Project Woman, a committee of the Oklahoma Division of the American Cancer Society which educates women about breast cancer. This story and the poem reflect a couple of Terry's more humorous adventures in her cancer experience.

First, I Cried
Bernie Beydler

"I was first diagnosed with breast cancer in 1976 during a routine breast exam by my regular doctor," stated Bernie Beydler. "He found a lump. I was sent for a mammogram and the finding was, yes, there was definitely something there." Bernie's husband recommended she see a breast cancer specialist. She underwent another mammogram and other examinations and had the lump biopsied. Her doctor later confirmed "it was definitely cancer," and said they would have to make arrangements for her to go to the hospital. "Lee was off doing engineering work and after the doctor got through talking to me, I sat down and I cried. I cried my eyes out. Then, I thought, 'That's kind of stupid.' My husband was gone doing consulting engineering work. I was his bookkeeper and nobody else was doing the work. I thought, 'darn, I was going to be out two or three weeks'; so I went back into my office and started working on the books so it would be okay while I was gone."

Bernie was worried how her husband would feel about her breast being removed. "He said, 'Honey, don't worry, you worry too much. You know I'm a leg man.' He was very, very helpful to me." Bernie had her left breast removed. In 1982, Bernie said she returned to the specialist because her right breast "had been feeling kind of funny." After being examined, "Sure enough, there was another lump there, deep into the breast." Bernie underwent a second mastectomy.

In 1986, Bernie felt another lump in her left breast and subsequently underwent a biopsy. Before she was placed under anesthetic, she asked the doctor, "How am I going to explain to my friends that I have had three mastectomies!" Bernie has a great attitude and sense of humor. She is now cancer free.

Bernie Beydler, age 75, of Heavener. Excerpts from an article written by Fran Johnson, Heavener Ledger, and submitted by Dee Ann Dickerson, Chair of the LeFlore County Women's Health Coalition in Poteau, Oklahoma. Bernie is a homemaker and retired bookkeeper in Heavener. She told her inspiring story at the April 1, 1995 Women's Health Forum in Poteau.

I'm Thankful
Suzie Eller

"Thank you Lord for another day." As I slip into my car to begin the morning of another busy day, I mentally give Him thanks for another healthy day. It has been three years and nine months since I was diagnosed with breast cancer and metastasis to the lymph nodes on my left side. When I meet people and they find out I had breast cancer, their reaction is always that of surprise. Just as I used to do, they picture a death sentence when cancer is pronounced. It is a battle, but not a death sentence.

"But do you know what the future holds?", I hear from well-meaning friends. I tell them that I know what today holds and I pray for what my future holds. By faith I will wake up and face my day with thanksgiving. I thank Him for my children… for my husband… for the flowers… for my job… for the teenagers in the youth group who said they would shave their heads to keep me company if I lost my hair… my sweet mother-in-law… the MRI that came back clear.

I'm thankful that I can still laugh about the hard things: the times I had to disrobe before an audience who did not understand my modesty; the laser show in the radiology lab; the technician who came in and began to feel my breast without identifying who he was and his reaction when I told him I wouldn't dare come in and feel a sensitive area of his body without telling him who I was and what I was doing. I'm thankful for the fact we still put plants in the office in my area because they seem to grow better now that I have had radiation (smile).

But most of all I'm thankful for His care. "I will never leave you or forsake you," the Bible says. Indeed, He never has.

Suzie Eller, age 35, of Muskogee. Suzie, a marketing coordinator for an engineering firm, was diagnosed at age 32. A wife, mother of three, youth sponsor, Sunday school teacher and discipleship leader for her church, Suzie uses one word to describe her life: busy. She feels breast cancer is not a death sentence. Because so many who get breast cancer do survive, she says adding faith to that number should improve the odds even more.

Get the Lead Out
Nancy Hane

I discovered the lump in my left breast the very evening after being taught how to do BSE (the correct way) by an American Cancer Society volunteer. I was 35 years old with a loving husband and two young children. My surgery and subsequent treatments were performed in Houston, where my brother and his family live. It was back in the days when a person was left in the hospital to recuperate. However, once out of the hospital, there were tests and then five days of chemo on my portable infusion pump. Altogether, I was away from home almost a month.

One sunny afternoon, while still in the hospital, a woman who worked for my brother visited me and asked if the Reach to Recovery volunteer had visited. When I said no, she went on to explain the program and that I would be given a temporary prosthesis made of fiberfill. She said that the prosthesis didn't weigh anything and that her experience was that it did not "hang" where the other breast "hung" and that it might also travel out of my bra and stick out of my shirt. Her solution to these problems was that Anne, my sister-in-law (later also diagnosed with breast cancer), and I should venture out to a sporting goods store and buy some lead fishing weights. Enough of these weights should be evenly dispersed among the fiberfill until the prosthesis weighed enough to "hang" where it would match my other breast and not float out of my bra.

The trip to the sporting goods store was uneventful except for a case of the giggles when a salesman asked if there was anything he could do to help us. We found the weights and fixed the prosthesis according to instructions. Tests were performed and the five days of chemo came and went. On the last day I was separated from the infusion pump. I gathered my belongings and we all headed for Hobby Airport and my return home. Not a thought was given to my prosthesis until—rounding the corner, I was faced with the metal detector! To this day, I remember turning and looking to my brother in utter panic. Amazingly, the detectors then were not sensitive enough to pick up the rather large lead fishing weights nestled securely in the fiberfill. While at that very moment it was not so funny, I now share this story with other women as an example of how to look back and laugh.

Nancy L. Hane, diagnosed in 1981 at age 35, now age 50, lives in Norman. A nurse since 1966, she became interested in oncology after her diagnosis, completing her BSN and Master's degrees; currently serves as an Oncology Nurse Clinician at INTEGRIS Baptist Medical Center. Focus of her life is marriage, raising two children and spreading the word about early detection of breast cancer. In giving something back to other women, Nancy is particularly proud of her work with the American Cancer Society project, "Circle of Life: A Breast Cancer Awareness Program for Native American Women."

Hang on to Humor
Nancy "Rosy" Glenn

I encourage you to practice awareness and early detection, for it could save your life. The words "breast cancer" should echo in every woman's mind to remind her to take charge by doing monthly self breast exams and having annual examinations and mammograms by her health care professionals.

And for all those survivors like me: don't forget humor. It's a must! For example, after losing all my hair within two weeks of starting chemotherapy, I decided to write a book on "101 Things to Do with a Fake Boob." (ha). On another occasion, one of my little neighbor buddies, five-year old Morgan, excitedly told his brother, "Rosy got really sick and sneezed and blew her hair off!"

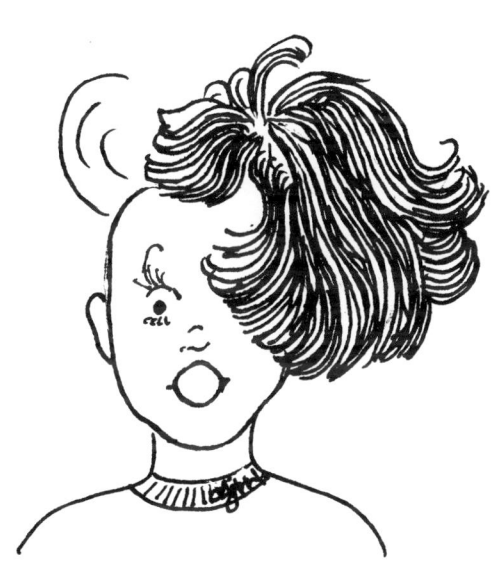

Nancy "Rosy" Glenn, age 39, of Tulsa.

Have Some Fun While You're Bald
Cindy Gibbs

Since being diagnosed with breast cancer, two events stand out in my mind as significant and special. The first occurred a few days before my biopsy when I was frightened and doubting God. I drove past a church building and noticed the message on the marquee; it was a scripture found in I Thessalonians 5:18. The verse says to "give thanks in all circumstances." My initial reaction was to snicker and think, "What in the world is there to be thankful for about having breast cancer?" I decided to give it a try and thanked God that evening for the circumstances I was facing and asked Him to help me find lessons to be thankful for. It was truly amazing to discover reasons for thankfulness over the next few weeks and to realize that breast cancer can be a blessing if I choose to make it one.

The second event occurred when my hair was falling out. I felt the tremendous need to make my hair loss a fun event for my children (ages 8, 4, and 1), so they could accept it more readily; therefore, I told them they could cut it off when the time came. The morning arrived and with much laughter and glee, they cut my hair to the scalp. For days they told their friends and mine that I was bald and they got to cut my hair. My daughter has had lots of fun showing my bald head to her friends at school and in our neighborhood and helping me choose which wig or scarf to wear. No one ever knows what to expect when they see me because I wear different colors and styles of wigs, hats and scarves. Hair loss has not been a problem for my children or me and I feel that the reason is because we made it FUN! My motto is, "If you have to be bald, you might as well have some fun while you're bald!"

Cindy Gibbs, age 38, of Oklahoma City. Cindy, diagnosed at 38, is a homemaker and mother. Her eight-year-old daughter, Laura, is a member of the Central Oklahoma Chapter of the Susan G. Komen Breast Cancer Foundation, Komen Kids™, a support group for children of loved ones who are suffering from life-threatening illnesses. Laura's account of this heartwarming experience and her responses to her mother's bout with breast cancer are presented on the following page.

Things Are Going Pretty Smooth
Laura Gibbs

On October 2nd, my mom had a mammogram. Two days later, she found out for sure she had breast cancer. In a few days, she had to have surgery. It was kind of cool going to the hospital. After that, people were bringing dinner to us and presents. Then, she had to start getting treatments at the hospital. She has to have six treatments. Now, she has to start taking medicine so that the treatments won't make her sick all the time. The chemotherapy made her lose her hair. When we were at my Grandma's house, she started losing her hair. She let my brother and me cut it off. We couldn't get the little hairs off, so my dad shaved her head with his shaver. It's a good thing she bought a wig!

Let me mention that the chemotherapy makes her really tired. It's not like she can't get up and do things. I haven't told you how I feel about this sickness. I really feel fine about it. The first time I saw the scar was at the hospital. After she lost her hair, it was neat playing in her wigs and things. I was not afraid to look at her head. To help me feel better, I go to a Counselor. I also go to a meeting. It's called Komen Kids™. Things are going pretty smooth. The end.

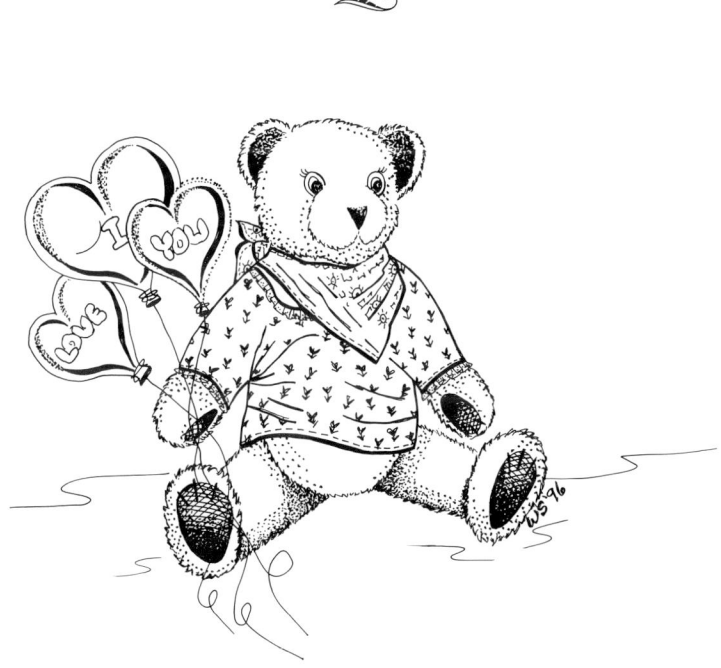

Laura Gibbs, age 8, of Oklahoma City, and daughter of Cindy Gibbs, is a member of the Komen Kids™, a support group for children of loved ones facing life-threatening illnesses, administered by the Central Oklahoma Chapter of the Susan G. Komen Breast Cancer Foundation.

5
Taking Care of Yourself
"We must take charge."

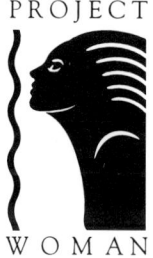

PROJECT

WOMAN

5
Taking Care of Yourself
"We must take charge."

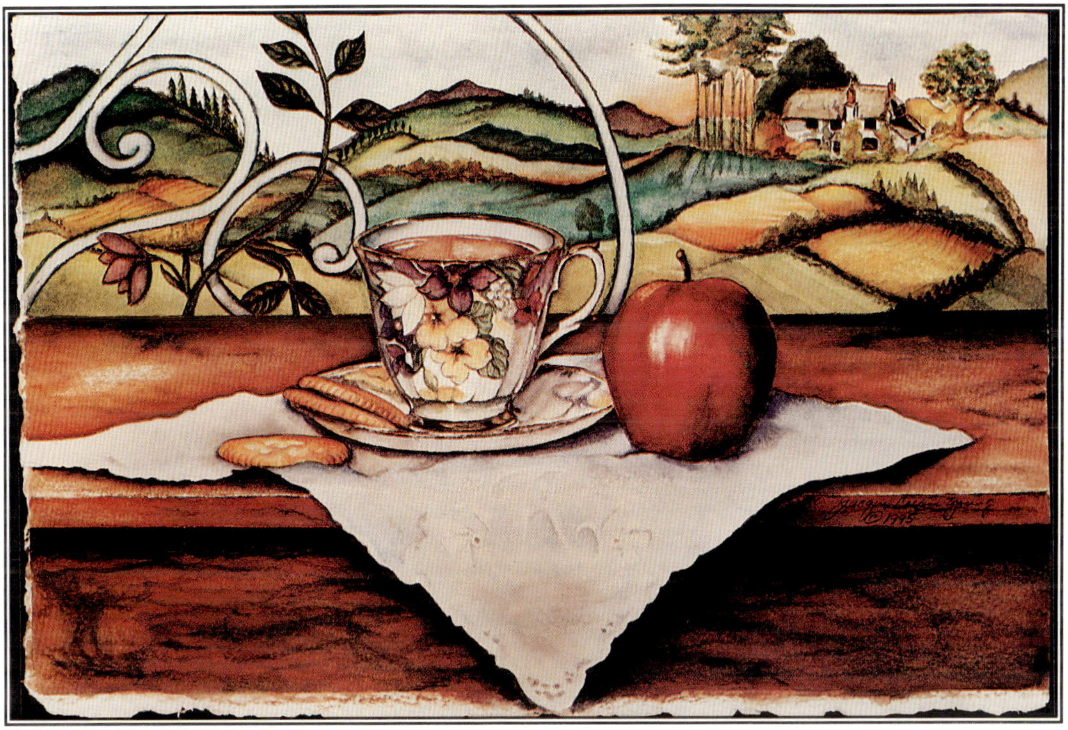

"Tea Thyme"   Jacque Collins Young

Jacque did this piece for a friend from England who is also a painter.

Take Charge of Your Body!
Joyce Elaine Hopson

I think my mother could have survived the battle of her life had she known the right questions to ask and actions to take before and after her diagnosis, states Amy Rudkins, daughter of Joyce Hopson. She could have sought different measures toward her treatment. Doctors have thousands of patients and they are not infallible; we should not expect them to be. Taking care of ourselves is our responsibility, no one else's. We should know our case history, study our medical records (they cannot be withheld from us), and seek second opinions when necessary.

My mother was not so lucky. She was a very brave woman with a gentle heart. She suffered more than I have ever seen any human suffer. She fought and fought, and finally accepted her fate in June 1990. She was only 39 years old. She had been married for 19 years and had one daughter, Amy (17) and a son, Beau (13).

We do not have to die! We must be educated about this horrible disease and be aware of all the decisions we face. Knowing the facts is so important to our treatment, recovery and ultimate survival. We must take charge of our bodies, our lives!

Joyce Elaine Hopson, of Hobart, died at age 39. Submitted in her memory by her daughter, Amy Rudkins. Joyce was diagnosed at age 35, when Amy was 12, and as a young woman, Amy lost her mother. She recalls that Joyce's life work was taking care of the people she loved—her family, friends and anyone in need, and Amy reminds us that we must do the same for ourselves.

My Crusade: Self-Exams! Mammograms
Verna Faye Wright

I don't know that my story is any different than others. My cancer was detected during my annual mammogram. They did a quadrantectomy on the breast, but did not check the lymph glands. My family and I felt it was necessary to know if the cancer had spread, so we sought a second opinion and another surgery. Radiation followed and soon I was back in the classroom and on a regular daily routine.

My crusade is self-examinations and regular mammograms! I nag, plead, and coerce. Also, never, never be afraid to get a second opinion and third opinion if necessary. Don't let a doctor or anyone else intimidate you. This is your life and your body.

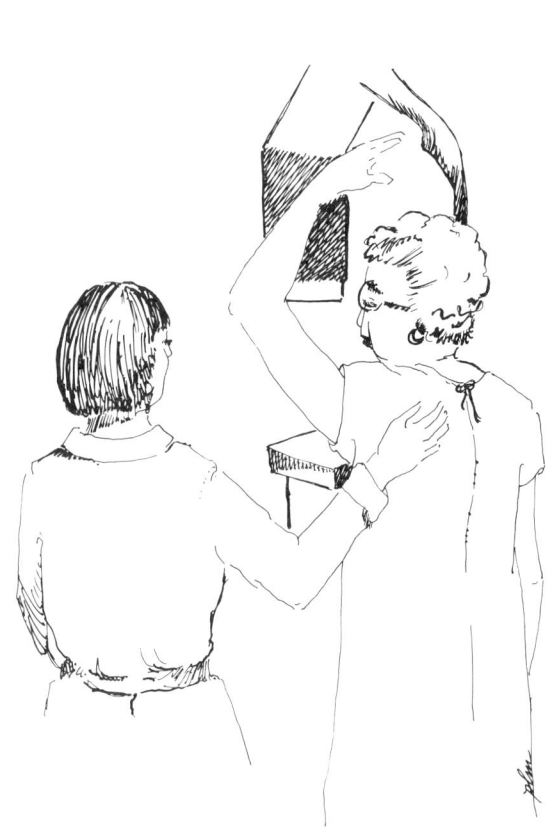

Verna Faye Wright, age 60, of Boise City. As both a school teacher and a Sunday school teacher, Verna knows the importance of a person's behavior. "Be careful what you do or say," she says. "You are someone's idol." Diagnosed at age 53, Verna has not let cancer defeat her. She still teaches school, serves on committees and square dances. A widow, Verna also keeps the yard mowed, the house painted, and the roof repaired.

I Know My Body Better
Susan Spencer

There has been no history of breast cancer in my family so I am not considered "high risk." Yearly gynecological visits which included breast exams have been a part of my routine, as well as monthly self-exams. In 1991, at age 37, I had a baseline mammogram which showed fibroid cysts in both breasts. Because breasts are dense in women under 50, it is difficult to see lesions or tumors on x-ray. My doctor said I probably didn't have anything to worry about.

When I turned 40, a surgeon examined me, compared past mammograms, consented to do a needle biopsy but felt that things were OK. I asked him to aspirate anyway and he found nothing. My longtime gynecologist agreed I had fibroid cysts that did not require surgery.

Yet, I knew my body better than any of them and I knew something was not right. I then made an appointment with a breast screening center. While I was informed that my insurance would probably not cover most of the testing, the extra cost was worth the peace of mind I needed. During the consultation, the female physician told me she was 90% certain I had cancer. After viewing each enhanced mammogram, the thermograms, the sonogram, the calcification groups, the tentacles from the cyst and three inflamed lymph nodes, I knew she was right.

On the next day the surgeon aspirated the tender spot and tests showed positive cancer cells. I had a complete mastectomy the following day. Three other physicians had examined me in the previous two months and saw nothing.

We must educate ourselves and save the lives of mothers and their daughters. In 1970, 1 out of 20 women had breast cancer. Today, 1 out of 8. My doctor predicts, by what she sees personally, in the year 2000 it will be 1 out of 3. That's getting pretty close to home.

Susan Spencer, age 41, of Idabel. Susan is a counselor for college students, abused children, and prisoners, and teaches college courses including criminal justice, psychology and sociology. She was diagnosed at age 40, and approaches life with cancer the same way as "how to eat an elephant—one bite at a time."

We Didn't Use the "C" Word
Thelma Ganes

~

When my great aunt and then my mother had breast cancer, you didn't talk about it. It was called a "malignancy." Saying CANCER was like using a four-letter word. But my mother taught me to examine myself and I became very aware of the importance of this procedure. Thank goodness the attitude about breast cancer is so different now!

~

Thelma Ganes, age 77, of Woodward. Submitted in her memory by her daughters, Debby Stine and Roxy Merklin. Thelma was a full-time wife and mother of three when she entered the retail business in 1967, eventually owning and operating a women's clothing store. She was first diagnosed at age 44, then again at age 53. She retired from her business in 1985, and was an active volunteer for the American Cancer Society and other community organizations.

Take Responsibility
Jessie Misner

~

Every woman who undergoes a mastectomy has a story to tell. It should be heard if she chooses to share it. My purpose is to tell the world there is life after breast surgery. Life is our most precious gift. Love your self enough to take personal responsibility for self-examination. Early detection and prompt treatment are the keynotes to survival.

~

Jessie Misner, age 75, of Sapulpa. Jessie, diagnosed at age 67, is a wife, mother and nurse practitioner with a local physician in an established family practice office. She is involved in numerous cancer-related organizations and projects, including the annual Creek County and Tulsa County Drive Against Breast Cancer.

Protect Our Future
Ertie Cook

~

Ertie's daughter, Donna Cook-Dragoo, recalls that her mother lost her own mother, sister, and niece to breast cancer, and finally her life as well. Donna added, "She had one sister and niece that are cancer survivors. She always had mammograms, physicals, and performed monthly self-exams. She was diagnosed with breast cancer twice in seven years, after locating each lump through self-examinations. My daughter, Angela, and I were inspired by her life and cautioned by her example to take responsibility for our breast care and protect our future."

~

Submitted by Donna Cook-Dragoo in memory of her mother, Ertie Cook, of Purcell. Ertie was first diagnosed at age 63 and then again at age 70. She was a restaurant owner for 30 years, but considered her life work to be a teacher's assistant. Ertie was always an active community volunteer for cancer-related organizations, Friends of the Library, adult reading, parent-teacher organization, and more.

Caring for the Caregiver
Lily Mae Cagle

This is a message for the caregivers. As a cancer survivor, I invite our society to become more cooperative toward the health and care of our women—mothers, wives, daughters, sisters and employees. Women need to be encouraged by family members, friends, and employers to give attention to their health before a crisis. It is proven that early detection of cancer, as was mine, saves many lives.

In particular, the woman who is a caregiver for a family member may often neglect her own welfare for the sake of another loved one. Or, the woman who is employed outside the home may not have her health care needs properly recognized by her family or the employer. In some instances, the demands of her caregiving responsibilities may cause her to forego her own needs; she may not even request leave from her employment for a few hours to seek health care.

Some of us are fortunate to have caring family members, friends, work associates and administrators. Not every woman is surrounded by such caring and cooperative people. We must take care of ourselves first of all, but sensitive awareness by others is necessary to help every woman detect breast cancer early.

Lily Mae Cagle, age 64, of Allen. Lily, a teacher of business education for 34 years in Oklahoma high schools, was diagnosed at age 54. Following her career in education, Lily worked for six years in the library at the Robert S. Kerr Environmental Research Laboratory in Ada. All during her professional career, she took care of her mother who had suffered a stroke at age 51. Married for 40 years, Lily has one daughter and two grandsons to whom she is a caregiver while her daughter works.

Like Thousands of Others
Nina Ritchie

I am a mother, grandmother, wife, daughter, and educator. And like thousands of other Oklahoma women, I am a cancer survivor. I had been divorced for more than ten years; then on December 15, 1991, I remarried. Six weeks later, I was diagnosed with cancer following a "suspicious" mammogram and biopsy. I underwent surgery, radiation, and chemo. My husband was with me all the way. Not only did I survive cancer but so did my marriage. Two of my maternal aunts died of breast cancer. They did not have the medical knowledge and expertise that were available to me, and they paid with their lives. I have great hope that future generations will have not just better treatments but a cure!

Nina Ritchie, age 45, of Poteau. A college educator, Nina was diagnosed at age 41. Her husband was with her through all phases of treatment and recovery.

Through Their Grief
Deborah Ann Gee

Debbie's life was taken by breast cancer at age 35. She was a wonderful daughter and a wonderful sister to her two brothers. She was always quick to help anyone in need. She left her mark on the community. Her church was made stronger. Her loss increased the public's awareness of breast cancer and its effects upon humanity. She left behind a husband and two small children. Through their grief possibly others can be made aware of this disease and death can be prevented through early detection.

Submitted by Virginia Weathers in memory of her daughter, Deborah Ann Gee, of Antlers. Debbie died at age 35, the same year she was diagnosed. A clerk for the Pushmataha County Health Department, Debbie was also a wife and mother of two small children. She was active in her church, played the piana and sang with a Christian singing group. Her mother remembers Debbie as a person always quick to help anyone in need, and she would regularly visit persons who were hospitalized and those in nursing homes.

Take Extra Precaution
Doris Calvert

"It's only knotted tissue and will never amount to anything." That diagnosis was wrong. In about six months, the lump began to throb and I became weak. So I returned to my doctor and within the week, I was without my breast.

So convinced was I that God would not allow this to happen to me, I did not prepare myself or my children. Mistake! To my sons, it was a death penalty; so little was known in 1976. For myself, it meant I would not return to work for a while and our finances suffered. Would my job still be there? Those were my worries, but I had a loving family, especially a husband who convinced me his love would not change.

My determination and faith in God kept me pushing to keep up the therapy and regain full use of my arm. My surgeon did not recommend radiation. Today, I would not take that chance, but would indeed take extra precaution.

Cancer could have wrecked my life, but I am thankful for my surgeon, my family and my church who were there for me.

Doris Calvert, age 65, of Pawnee. Doris was diagnosed at age 45, has been the wife of a pastor for 25 years, a bookkeeper for 20 years, and the co-caretaker of a Baptist camp for five years. She has devoted her life to ministry and service to other people through her many roles in the church. She accompanies her husband on literally hundreds of home, hospital, and nursing home visits each year.

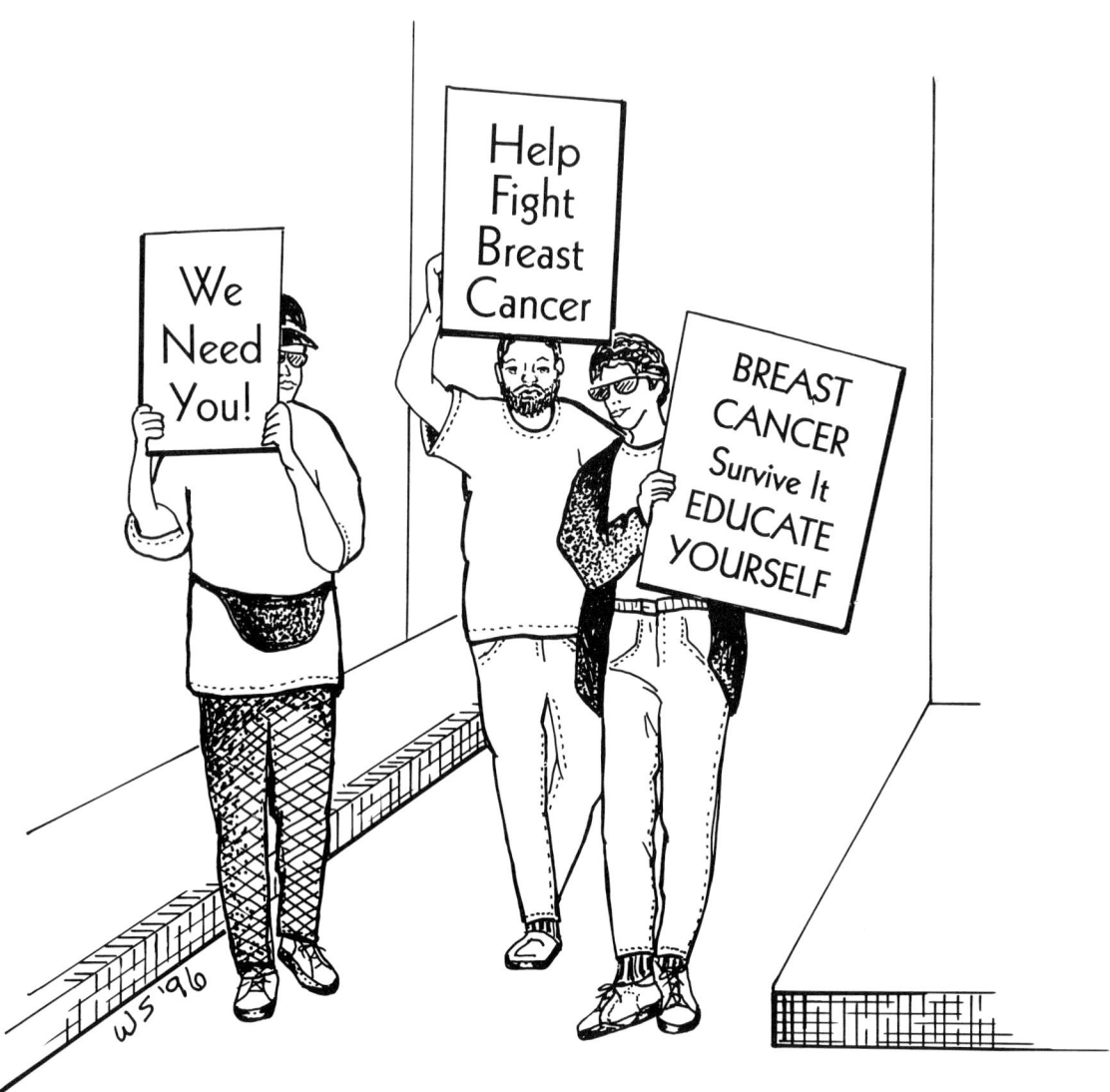

Borrowed Time
Peggy L. Funk

Peggy Funk, a registered Delaware Indian, was born in 1950 in Vinita, Oklahoma, and grew up in Sand Springs. She was stricken with inflammatory breast cancer in August 1989, and was sent home to die. Peggy not only began her fight with the disease she encountered, she also fought the apathy that surrounds the issue. She became an active lobbyist at the national, state and county levels for breast cancer awareness, research and cure. Peggy declared: "I'm on borrowed time, and I refuse to pass on this legacy of NO CAUSE, NO PREVENTION, NO CURE to my daughter and granddaughter!" Reporter Juliann Smith observed that despite the disease returning and wreaking havoc on her system, "Funk managed to find the energy to rise every morning and put her own pain aside to fight so that others after her will not have to go through what she has gone through."

In 1993, Peggy received a proclamation from Governor Pete Wilson (CA) and the state assembly for her efforts which effectively brought about the passage of AB478, which put a two-cent tax on cigarettes for breast cancer research and detection. She "cajoled, pleaded and explained the long overdue need of Americans to stop looking at breast cancer as a personal tragedy but as a horrible epidemic." Her admonitions to all women are, "Be an assertive patient. Get options, get answers. Stay informed on federal and state issues affecting breast cancer. Know where your legislators stand and if they are supportive. If they are not supportive, vote them out!"

In October 1993, Peggy's daughter, Lori Loud of Tulsa, accepted a Salute to Women award on her mother's behalf. Peggy Funk was one of 12 women who were recognized for their exceptional contributions in Ventura County, CA. Lori passed on her activist mother's plea for cancer patients to stop being helpless and to take action. Her concluding remarks at the awards banquet were, "Mom would like to offer hope and a prayer to each one of you—that you won't be diagnosed with breast cancer." Peggy's daily affirmation was taken from Jeremiah 30:17, "I will restore your health and heal your wounds."

Submitted by Lori Loud, of Tulsa, in memory of her mother, Peggy Funk, who died at age 44. Excerpts also included from article by staff writer Juliann Smith, The Fillmore Gazette (CA), October 13, 1993. Peggy, diagnosed at age 41, had moved to California to take part in an experimental cancer drug study. After a long and courageous campaign to raise awareness about breast cancer at state and national levels, Peggy received a proclamation from California Governor Pete Wilson for those efforts, and was invited to meet with First Lady Hillary Rodham Clinton to give her thoughts on health care.

I Got to Know My Mom
Peggy J. Smith

I am one of seven children, third down the line among five girls and two boys. I still cry when I think about my mom. The one-year anniversary of her death just came and went. I don't know when it will get better, when it will get easier to talk about, but I'm told it will. My mom was so vibrant and so full of life that it made you tired just watching her go. She was a beautiful woman. She had blond hair, sparkling blue eyes and a dazzling smile for everyone. She had a quick wit, enjoyed making fun of herself, and she was always laughing. That's the way she was before cancer.

Mom was first diagnosed in 1990. She found a lump in her breast, about three centimeters in size. She wanted the cancer to be gone, so she chose to have her breast removed. She had no follow-up treatment. In June 1993, after months of coughing and difficulty in breathing, she discovered that cancer had returned with a vengeance. Mom was so scared. After months of chemotherapy and maximum radiation treatments, she was miserable. She had gone from 180 lbs. to over 200 lbs. of puffiness. Her hair was gone; her head, chest, and back had raw blisters from the radiation. She wanted to quit. She said, "The cure is worse than the kill." I begged her to continue. I thought that I could give her the strength she needed. I tried to be her shield. I was learning about her and fighting for her. I tried to soften the blows. But it was her fight and she was losing.

Throughout her illness, Mom spent a lot of time talking to my sisters and me about breast cancer awareness. She wanted us to be aware of our bodies as she had not been. Together, we became two of the founding members and board of directors for the Central Oklahoma Chapter of the Susan G. Komen Breast Cancer Foundation. She got involved as much as her illness would allow. We lost her the day following our inaugural running of the Race for the Cure, a race to raise funds for local breast cancer projects. My sisters and I hope to help others become aware of breast cancer and the importance of early detection of this disease.

June 1993 through June 1994 was a difficult year for me. There was a lot of pain, a lot of grief and a lot that I wish I hadn't had to go through. It was also the year that I got to know my mom.

Submitted by Darla Buckner, one of five daughters and two sons, in memory of their mother, Peggy Smith, of Moore. Peggy was diagnosed at age 50 and died at age 54. She was a homemaker and owner/operator of a catering shop. She was on the founding board of directors for the Central Oklahoma Chapter of the Susan G. Komen Breast Cancer Foundation, and was devoted to increasing awareness of the importance of early detection.

God's Not Through with Me Yet!
Betty Laura Channell

～

Betty was a very vital person who enjoyed life, always had a smile and loved to make people laugh. When she was 53 years old, she discovered a problem in her right breast during self-examination. She promptly made an appointment with her physician who performed a biopsy and diagnosed the cancer. Doctors advised her that seven out of ten nodes were malignant. She then had the breast removed, followed by the maximum treatment prescribed. Although the treatments made her deathly ill, Betty continued to have her upbeat personality and encouraged her family that she would beat the illness. Moreover, she encouraged every woman she visited with to have a yearly mammogram and to check her breasts every month. Because of her influence, all her sisters and daughters religiously have physical exams and mammograms and do monthly breast exams. Her vigilance led her to discover an area where the skin was puckered from a pulling within her breast. She notified her doctor immediately, and the results no doubt helped to extend her life an additional 20 years. Her cancer never returned; Mom died of a stroke when she was 74. And to the very end she would say, "Hey, I'm still living! That means God's not through with me yet!"

～

Submitted by Letha Clark in memory of her mother, Betty Channell, of Tishomingo. Betty was diagnosed with breast cancer at age 53, and died of stroke at age 74. Betty was a recruiter for a Convair aircraft plant in California during World War II to search for women to help build the B-32, Dominator super bombers and other war planes; after the war she moved back to Johnston County to be with her family and became a partner in the family business, Channell Butane and Plumbing, until 1966, at which time she moved to Norman, went back to school, became a lab technician and worked for the mental hospital lab. Her "spare" time led her to develop a musical organization of Tishomingo business leaders, called the Okie Nitwits, that performed for the Red Cross and other non-profit organizations to raise money.

6
Care and Support from Others
"That's okay, we'll take care of it."

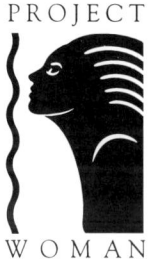

6
Care and Support from Others
"That's okay, we'll take care of it."

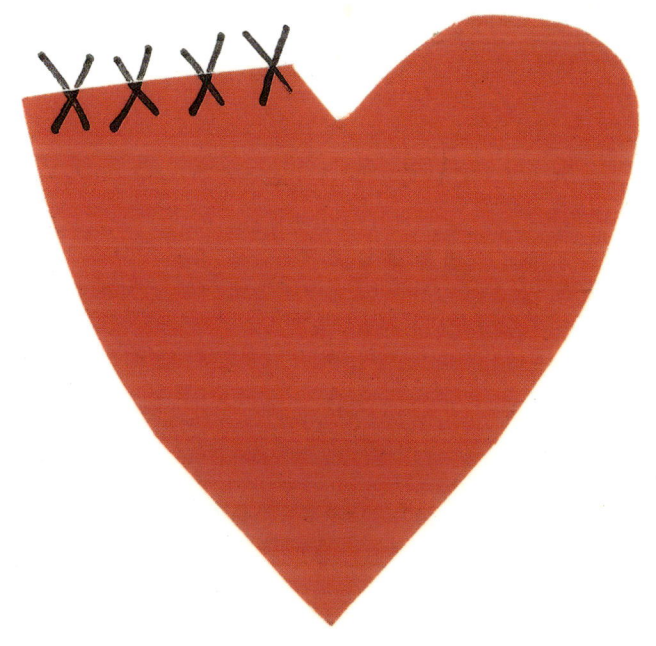

Valentine with an attitude

In memory of my left breast removed 12/21/92. On with chemotherapy

"Valentine with an attitude" Margie Needham

Margie Needham is a graphic artist, a children's art teacher, and she is a breast cancer survivor. This piece is a media collage which, she says, she "sent as a postcard to friends, family, and medical personnel who helped me through surgery." A photograph of Margie and a poem by her friend, John Brandenburg, are found on pages 104-105.

That's Okay, We'll Take Care of It
Charlotta Atwell

It's the last week of February, 1990. My best friend and I are attending a week-long critical care course in Oklahoma City; we both are RNs. After a tiring day of driving to and from the course in addition to a full day of lectures, I'm more than ready for my bed. As I lie there, allowing my body to relax from the day's tensions, I casually run a hand over my left breast. Wait! What was that? I feel it again and, yes, there it is again, a lump. I try desperately to control my panic. When Terry, my husband of 22 years, slides into bed next to me, I confide my greatest fear. He feels it too, but is quick to encourage me not to jump to conclusions. I'm a nurse. I know all the possibilities. I finally agree with him to control my emotions and take the next logical step—check it out with the doctor.

I made the appointment for March 7th. A biopsy was scheduled for March 9th. The doctor felt there was no cause for alarm, but as a precaution the tissue was sent to pathology. Now it's Wednesday, March 14th. I haven't heard anything from the reports. We 've just finished dinner when the phone rings. It's the doctor, "I have some bad news. It's cancer." My son had come into the room while I was on the phone and could tell something was wrong, so he went to get his dad. As I hung up the phone, I turned to them and said, "I have breast cancer." I had said it out loud and the full impact suddenly hit me. As I nearly dropped to the floor, my husband grabbed me and said, "That's okay, we'll take care of it." That statement became our motto over the next few months. It became a team effort.

I was scheduled for a mastectomy on March 26th. I was a patient in my own hospital; no longer the nurse giving care, but receiving it. My co-workers were great. They were all supportive and optimistic, which made everything easier to deal with. Times got rough over the next few months, but through it all, we said, "That's okay, we'll take care of it."

Now it's 1995. I'm still working the 11-7 shift as House Supervisor. My son is following in my footsteps, currently attending LPN school. My daughter plans the same in the near future. My husband is still beside me through everything, and there have been some scares, but he is always there to say, "That's okay, we'll take care of it."

Charlotta Atwell, age 45, of Ninnekah. Charlotta, a registered nurse, was diagnosed at age 40, and currently works as the house supervisor at Grady Memorial Hospital in Chickasha. In addition to her work as a nurse, she enjoys babysitting three active grandchildren, doing counted cross stitch, camping and hosting family gatherings.

Community Property
Lynn Witzen

At the age of 38 I was an independent career woman. I worked hard to balance my career, care for a home and participate in church and volunteer activities. I remember our minister explaining one Sunday that challenges in our lives can be opportunities for growth. Little did I know that I would encounter such a giant opportunity that year.

My life came to a screeching halt when I was diagnosed with breast cancer. All those activities that were so important now seemed quite trivial. I was in a life or death struggle. I had to find a way to cope with the crises that would face me in the months ahead.

First off, it was a real challenge for me to ask for and accept help from others. I know how often I wanted to do things for friends who faced difficulties. Now, here I was in the midst of my own dilemma. My friends readily offered their assistance, but it was a struggle for me to let go of my sense of independence.

After soul searching and prayer, I reached a moment of understanding: A community of friends is not a group of individuals independent of one another. A community is interdependent, where the roles of helper and being helped are interchangeable. At that moment, I let go, gratefully accepting help from others. Yes, I was willing to be "community property." It was an incredible feeling of love and acceptance when I could say, "I'm really scared," and receive the support and understanding of friends. There were messages of encouragement, affirming my faith, my will to live, and a reminder of my commitment to invest in my life.

My minister was right. This challenge was filled with opportunities. The victory of life isn't mine alone. It is shared with the many friends who supported me along the way. It feels kind of nice to be "community property."

Lynn Witzen, age 40, of Stillwater. Lynn was diagnosed at age 38, and has spent her professional career as a registered occupational therapist helping people with neurological problems. She works in home health care and has also worked for a host of volunteer activities, including serving as a Special Olympics coach.

Linda's Love Team
Linda Kirkpatrick

This story is not only about me, a breast cancer survivor, but also about a special group of people who have built unique relationships with each other and the bonding that has taken place. It all began on New Year's weekend 1994. "You have a cancerous lump in your breast and it must come out immediately." I looked at the radiologist stunned; I was numb and couldn't move. Finally, I left the office to go back to work thinking, "What on earth do I do now?" After talking with my gynecologist, I visited a surgeon and in two days the lump was taken out. Later results of blood tests indicated the cancer had spread to my liver and that I must undergo ten months of chemotherapy. But, I knew I could lick this and become healthy again. So a plan of action began.

For over a year a group of ten members of my church and I had been doing aerobics together. Upon hearing the news, they soon started a support group. A T-shirt was created showing a big yellow smiling sunshine face on the front and on the back was "Linda's Love Team." We met once each month for supper, laughter, and loving fellowship. They were always there when I needed them. Together, with my family and twin sister, everyone kept me on the right track. I never thought I was doomed.

Today, I am healthy and have more energy than ever. Life is so fragile and precious; I take one day at a time and live it to the fullest. I am deeply indebted to my family, my sister, and my "Linda's Love Team." My desire now is to help others who undergo this challenge and tell them, "You can make it, too."

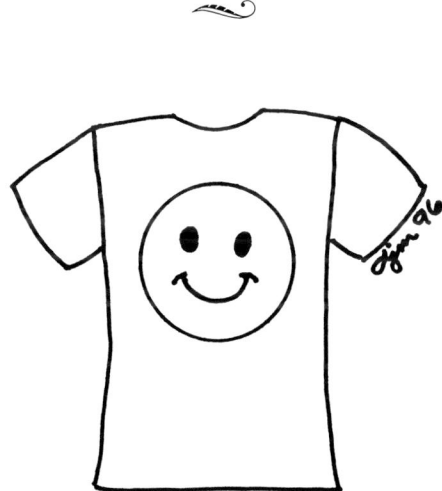

Linda Kirkpatrick, age 55, of Oklahoma City. Linda was diagnosed at age 54. After teaching fifth grade in the Midwest City-Del City school system for four years, she devotes her life to raising her two children and serving faithfully in various capacities on the administrative staff at St. Luke's United Methodist Church.

The Mountain Top
Carol Bond Parker

My faith in God and a very loving family helped me live through cancer. My sisters, son, and sister-in-law took me for my treatments. They sat with me when I threw up, drove me to ball games (I'm a girl's basketball coach) when I was too sick, emptied the foul smelling trash cans and aired out the house after the treatments. They loved me when I was most unlovable.

My daughters and son had to see me cry when my hair came out. They endured the tremendous mood swings due to hormonal imbalance. They witnessed all my human frailties because I was brought to the brink of death while trying to get well. But my hair grew back even nicer. My health gradually came back to normal. I moved to a better job. And, a wonderful man came into my life and he is now my husband.

After the valley of the shadow of death, God allowed me to see the mountain top.

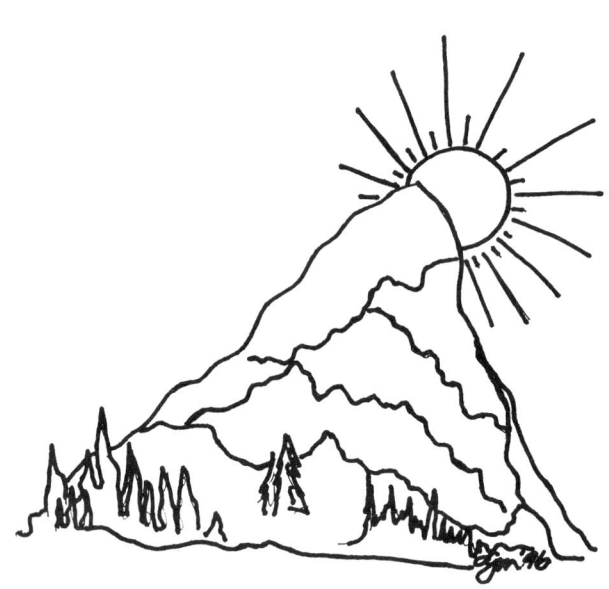

Carol Bond Parker, age 46, of Cashion. A mother of three, Carol was diagnosed at age 40, soon after she had accepted a position to coach high school girl's basketball and to teach English in Morris, Oklahoma. A former all-state and all-decade basketball player in her own right, Carol wants to teach women that breast cancer can affect women of all ages.

Kindness Even from Strangers
Maryl Thomas-Griffitts

I am a breast cancer survivor. I was first diagnosed at the age of 37; my son was only two years old. I will never forget that moment. It was devastating. I kept remembering my father's death from lung cancer, not even a year earlier. Previously, I had been refused a mammogram because I was too young and there was no history of breast cancer in my family.

I had a modified mastectomy with immediate reconstructive surgery. The costs were staggering and the battles with the insurance company were endless. But through it all, the care and support were always there—from loved ones and friends, from medical staff and co-workers. I am extremely fortunate to have had the kindness and generosity of so many people, some of whom I'd never met.

They mailed get-well cards, placed my name on prayer lists, sent flowers and plants, gave gifts and money throughout my illness and recovery. At Christmas, I was undergoing chemotherapy treatments. I was not able to be out among the crowds because my immune system was compromised. The wonderful people I work with surprised me with toys, food, gift certificates and money for our Christmas and medical expenses. The women in my mother's church group collected food for our Christmas. Even the firm where I was employed increased my life insurance and gave me a raise in salary. Never have I felt such unselfish kindness and love. Words can never express my sincere gratitude.

Maryl Thomas-Griffitts, age 41, of Oklahoma City. An accountant who specializes in income tax preparation, Maryl was diagnosed at age 37. She is very open about discussing her illness, and has the ability to see humor even in an illness as grave as breast cancer.

Another Healing
Roseanna D. Smith

I danced, I laughed, I cried.

I sang, I touched, I loved.

My body was rocked and cradled and rocked
    from somewhere deep within me
    came memories of earlier, infant love.

I heard the humming
    as my tears flowed
    to cleanse my soul.

Pictures were drawn, studied,
    shared glimpses of a five-year-old
    gained clarity and understanding.

And with the insight came more forgiving
    more letting go
    letting go into love.

Affirmations became bonds, a joining of
    differing spirits into one
    deeply sharing, opening to glorious trust.

I was ocean, I was seaweed.

Gentle fingers brushed my branches,
    softening bellies
    opening hearts

Reaching deeply into parts before unclaimed.

Roseanna D. Smith, age 53, of Oklahoma City. Roseanna wrote this poem during her recovery from breast cancer. She dedicates the poem to her mother, Geraldine Nelson, who died of breast cancer in 1981. Roseanna, a Licensed Marriage and Family Therapist in Oklahoma City, was diagnosed in 1990 at age 49.

Another Healing Revisited
Val Ray

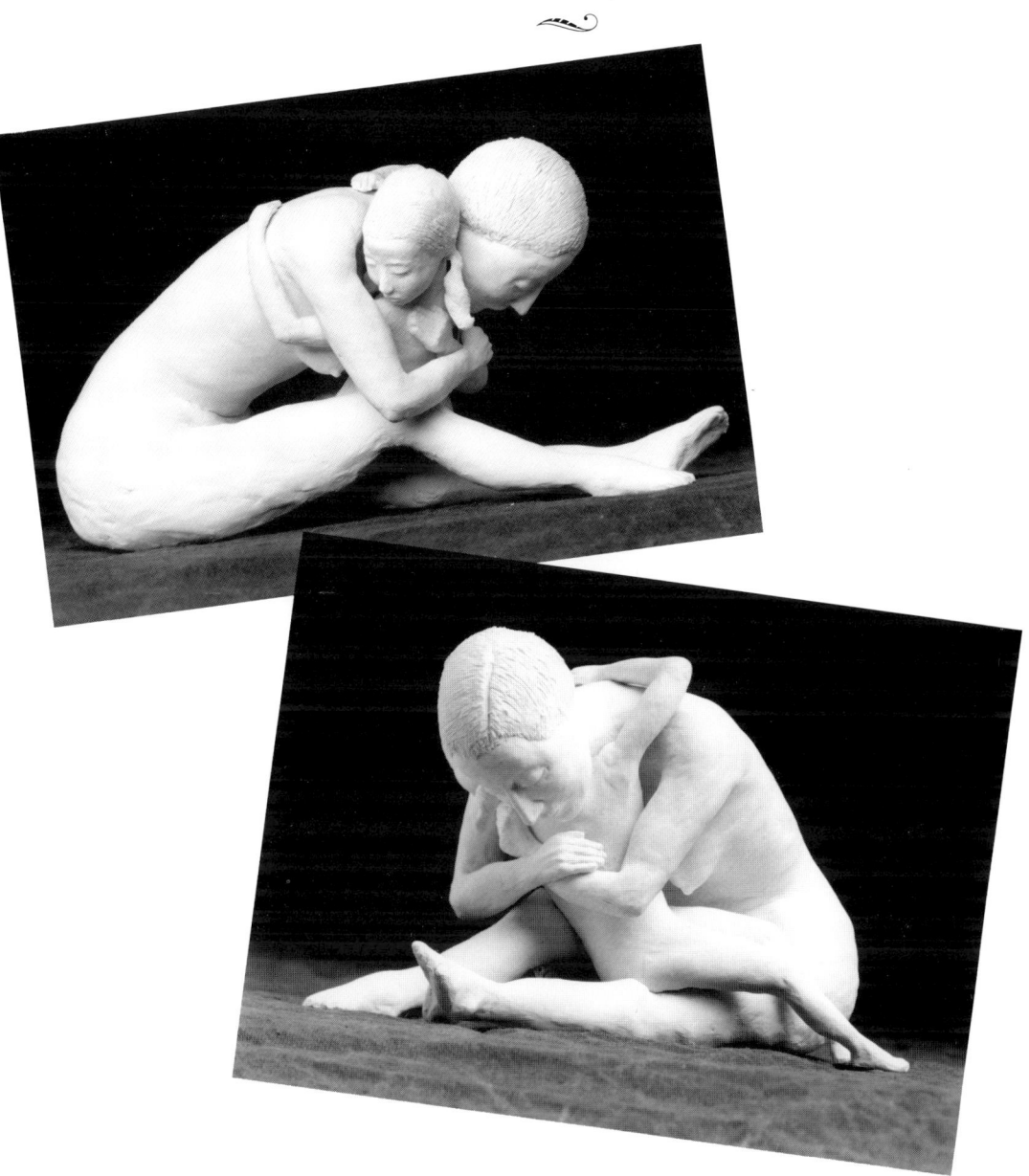

The photographs above depict the sculpture on the cover page entitled, Another Healing Revisited, *by Val Ray. Val was inspired to create the sculpture upon reading the preceding poem,* Another Healing, *by her friend, Roseanna Smith. According to Val, "One day Roseanna was sharing her experiences with breast cancer and she read her poem to me. A profound sense of 'her truth,' as she calls it, rippled through me. It was a sacred moment. I felt this overwhelming passion to create the sculpture. I believe that healing in all its forms represents rebirth, a renewal of the body or that of one's mind and spirit. To that end, I dedicate this sculpture to my friend, Roseanna Smith."*

Sisterhood of Survivors
Maggie Casto

I'm an important statistic: I'm one of the "one in nine" women predicted to get breast cancer in their lifetime. Now, through the sisterhood of survivors, I have discovered there is life after breast cancer. Everywhere I turned, I received encouragment. Jo C. shared pictures of her bicycle ride across the USA two years after her mastectomy. My next door neighbor told me about her mother's lumpectomy years ago. My sister-in-law autographed a copy of the book she wrote after surgery. The volunteer from Reach to Recovery came out and listened to me, then shared her experiences. Another neighbor merely gave me a hug and said, "I've been there, too. Twice." Even the friends who did not survive gave me, while they were still alive, the love, courage, and support that can come only from someone who has walked a mile in your shoes.

These friends all reminded me that I had a second chance. Life had not been taken away from me, after all; merely changed. I lost a breast, a body part. That body part does not define who I am. The loss doesn't prevent me from riding my bicycle or quilting or writing. It doesn't keep me from enjoying friends or worshiping God or serving others. It most certainly doesn't keep me from loving or being loved by my husband. And it didn't affect my sense of humor. As I told my surgeon, now I can hit the half-off lingerie sales. I just hope it's not the wrong half off.

None of us is given a guarantee of the number of years we will have. **Today** is what we have; tomorrow is what we hope for. As Dolly told her brothers in Bill Keane's cartoon, *Family Circus*, "Today is a gift from God. That's why it's called the present." With the support of the sisterhood of survivors and the love of family and friends, I'm unwrapping my beautiful present day by day.

Maggie Casto, age 53, of Tulsa. Maggie was diagnosed at age 51. She is a wife, mother, friend, and writer, leading an active life covering church and personal activities. She enjoys people and places, especially those places filled with wildflowers and birds. As a writer, Maggie has expressed in words her personal experience with breast cancer.

You Can't Do It by Yourself
Sharon Petrik

During chemotherapy I began losing my hair. I then debated whether to get a wig or try hats. Tony, my husband, liked the way I look in hats. Now I wear them all the time. It's my trademark.

Surviving cancer is with me every day. So many people have helped me. The support from the family and talking with others is so very important. That is the value of support groups. We can look around the room and know every woman has had breast cancer and they have gone on with their lives. We share stories, cry, and hug. We give lots of hugs. Studies have shown that women who participate in support groups survive better.

Dealing with breast cancer is hard work. You can't do it by yourself. Your shoulders are not that broad. But my faith and a smile and laugh are with me each day. And a hell of sense of humor doesn't hurt. I get a kick out of life! Hey, where's my hat?

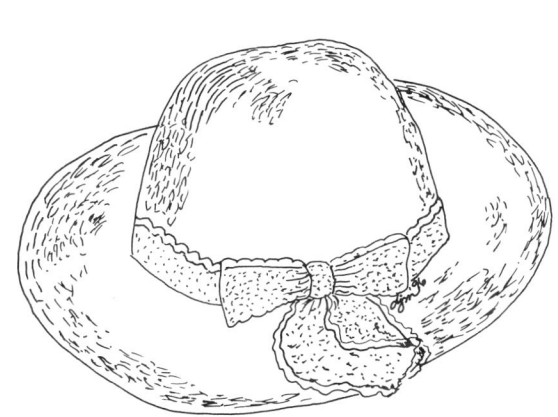

Sharon Petrik, age 45, of Broken Arrow. Submitted by her daughter, Kay Petrik. Sharon, who was diagnosed at age 43, owns Petrik Drug and Soda Fountain along with her husband, Tony. She organized a breast cancer support group in Broken Arrow and has been active in various cancer-related organizations. Portions of this tribute are courtesy of an article which appeared in the Broken Arrow Ledger.

Their Turn to Give Back
Lori Bennitt

It was just a routine biopsy to remove another benign tumor, or so we thought. But cancer had struck our family again. Our mother had died of breast cancer and was diagnosed in the early stages just as Lori's was this time. The two weeks that followed Lori's diagnosis were filled with difficulties and anxiety. Her husband relived the painful deaths of his own mother and mother-in-law at the hands of this monster. Following consultations, the doctors all came to the same conclusion, given Lori's family history—remove both breasts and start chemotherapy right away. Being a strong and courageous person, she didn't want to waste a moment. But as the gurney rolled in, I will never forget her words, "I had no idea what mom was going through 'til now. No one can ever imagine."

The effects of the radical mastectomy and chemotherapy were devastating. We had watched our mother endure her physical battle with cancer; now through our sister's eyes we witnessed the emotional battle, but we would never fully understand the fear and pain she experienced. Yet, through her sense of loss of her femininity, her loss of hair and countless other side effects, Lori always had a smile and deep concern for others first.

The sister I have always admired and envied as a generous giver was now in need of our love and support. We have a wonderful, close family, but who would have expected that her small town neighbors would bring in hot meals daily for the next several months. All those folks who brought food to Lori's door said it was "their turn to give back" to this totally unselfish person as she had always done for them.

Lori Bennitt, age 38, of Hobart. Submitted by her sister, Liz Poole. Lori was diagnosed at age 37, is a wife and mother of two boys. She is a secretary at the elementary school in Hobart, a Girl Scout leader, Boy Scout leader and Sunday school teacher. Lori and Liz's mother, Lynn Ensz, died from breast cancer.

Let Friends Help
Deborah Nevels

You are able to see the love everyone has for you when you are in a situation like this. My family did all they could and my friends did the rest. It really makes you feel comforted. I attend a support group. It is amazing how this group helps me. I have decided to reach out to any woman who has to go through the same ordeal. You know then you are not alone. Don't be afraid to let your friends help you.

Deborah Nevels, age 40, of Elk City. Diagnosed at age 39, Deborah works for Meridian Oil as an operations assistant. She is very active with her family and the First Baptist Church, as well as summer youth baseball and girl's softball.

Life Is Good
Marcia M. Tosee

It all began in October 1987. My youngest daughter was sitting on my lap and accidentally elbowed my breast. It got sore but I passed it off as a bruise, then I noticed a lump. Surgery was done and my life was forever changed. It all happened so fast. My oldest daughter kept things going around the house and my son helped with the chores outside. My husband stood by my side good days and bad. I am a very lucky woman. It is going on nine years since that fateful October. I now have four grandkids, and I can't explain how precious their lives are to me. Life is good and it can be taken away in a heartbeat. The most beautiful things in the world cannot be seen or touched, but are felt in the heart.

Marcia Tosee, age 42, of Waurika. Marcia, diagnosed at age 34, is a very special person according to her husband, Pepper. She is special not only to him, but also to her daughter, the rest of her family and all the people she meets. Marcia feels her survival means there is life after cancer, and she would like to give other people hope no matter how dim it looks at times.

From the Mouths of Babes
Lawana Giddings

I am the youngest child and only girl among four children. I married a wonderful man who continued to cushion me in life's difficulties. But I knew this was my cross alone; no one else could do it for me. I thought I had faced the worst of it, then the doctor told me that after treatments I would lose my hair. I was numb. It felt urgent to contact my daughter who was away in college. I called her and she came home immediately. As we were backing out of the driveway, I said, "Jill, my hair is beginning to come out real fast, so the next time you see me I will be wearing a wig." She stopped the car and with tear-filled eyes she said, "Mom, it's the kind of mom you are that matters, not your hair." God blessed me through my child.

Lawana Giddings, age 46, of Okmulgee. An office manager for State Farm Insurance, she is involved in many community organizations. One of her favorites is CASA Program. She also serves as a Safehouse board member and has been the fundraising chair. Diagnosed at age 45, Lawana is determined to return to a fun life.

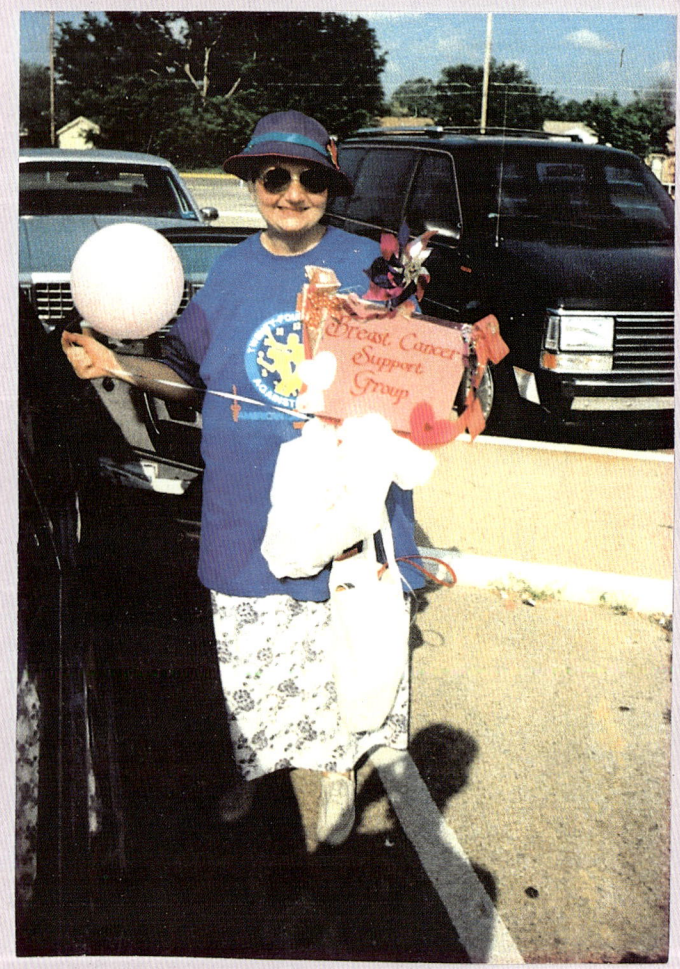

Margie Needham

Morning
Margie Needham

A lavender morning quietly dawns.
I hear Margie sneeze in her room.
Once, twice, but she sounds all right.
I sleep another few minutes.
Lavender giving way to grey skies.
Overcast.
When will they clear?
Bandaged.
Sewn together with branches.
On the third day of the year.

Poem and photograph by John Brandenburg, friend of Margie Needham, age 57, of Norman. Margie, who was 54 when she was diagnosed, is a graphic artist and children's art teacher.

From Hell to Heaven with Man's Best Friend
Janice Lea Bingaman

Saying goodbye for the last time is the hardest thing I will ever do in my life. As I look back on my life with Duke, my tiny five-pound Yorkshire Terrier, my soul smiles remembering the special times we shared as well as the ordinary, everyday things that were made special by having this little dog share my life. Having cancer is never easy, but being single I missed the emotional and physical support of having a spouse or children nearby at this most crucial time. Duke and I had lived alone together for eight years, and he was constantly at my side, napping in my lap or snuggled under the covers sleeping peacefully against my back. With all my relatives living in another state and my friends consumed with their work, I relied on my little furry companion to be more than just a dog.

Some ancient religions believed that dogs were sent here to take care of us, rather than us taking care of them. I feel certain that God sent Duke to take care of me. He comforted me in those most difficult times of chemo, radiation and chronic fatigue syndrome, never wavering in his commitment or unconditional love. He was the only one who never left my side. I think of Duke as an old mystic soul. He epitomized the fundamental characteristic of understanding God's purpose and the true meaning of life—to give and accept love. How strange that this most human of emotions has been expressed so perfectly by my not-quite-human friend.

Duke is a dog hero. Oh, I know that he never saved anyone from a burning building, pushed a wheelchair or led the blind, but Duke took care of me through the fear, pain, and loneliness of cancer, giving love and asking nothing but my presence in return. Like an angel watching over me, he rested quietly by my side, forsaking earthly treasures like food and play, feeling the beat of my heart as I slept, and promising never to leave me no matter where my journey took me. How unfortunate that dogs, like people, are often valued more by what they do instead of who they are.

What a strange quirk of fate that a few months ago the tables were turned when Duke was diagnosed with kidney and heart failure. I now found myself the caretaker, watching over him at death's doorstep. Only then did I understand the helplessness that a caretaker feels, wanting their loved one just to be well again, while knowing it can never be. How terrified Duke must have been watching me endure endless days of illness as cancer and chemo sucked the life out of me. How hard it must have been for this little dog, as I slept for days without awakening, pricked by the poison spinning wheel of Cytoxan. Sometimes, when I was only partly awake, I would catch him stealing my breath with his nose pressed close to mine, making sure I was still alive. Now I wondered if he would ever lick my face again, just as he must have wondered if I would ever waken to pet his head or cradle him in my lap.

I drove Duke to the hospital, crying out loud to him to hang on and not die, as I watched his tiny body stiffen in agonizing pain. With his teeth clenched and trembling and his eyes barely conscious, I saw him look at me through the pain, ruggedly determined to obey his master's final request. I visited Duke in the hospital each day, spending hours talking and reminiscing, trying to make sure that nothing was left unsaid. I prayed for him to be cured, but it was not to be.

I always believed it was I who was supposed to die first. I would leave this world from my own bed, surrounded by family and friends, with Duke nestled closely at my side. Instead, I did for him what I knew he would do for me. I brought him home from the hospital for one last time. I invited our friends to be present as we all said goodbye. And then, in a special ceremony surrounded by those who loved him, I let him go. He was wrapped in a hand-made flannel blanket, placed in a cotton quilt-lined wooden box and buried under my bedroom window where he could keep watch over me.

Because I believe so much that Duke was sent here to take care of me, I also believe, as our forefathers believed, that our dogs go on to heaven before us to show us the way. Heaven could not exist for me if Duke were not there; so I trust that he is an angel looking down on me, patiently waiting for his master to come home. And when my days on earth are done, I know he will once again eagerly greet me and, making sure I don't get lost along the way, he will gently lead me on the road to heaven.

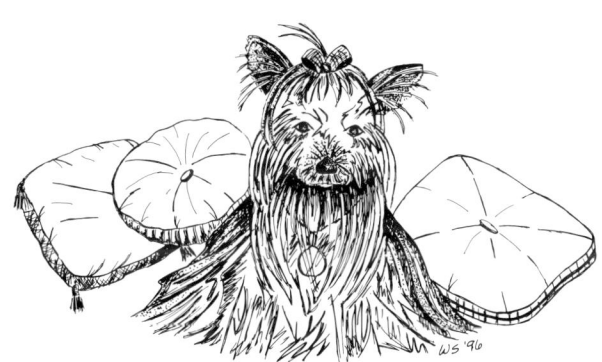

Janice Bingaman, age 41, of Oklahoma City. Janice was 38 when she was diagnosed, and was formerly a senior professional pharmaceutical sales representative.

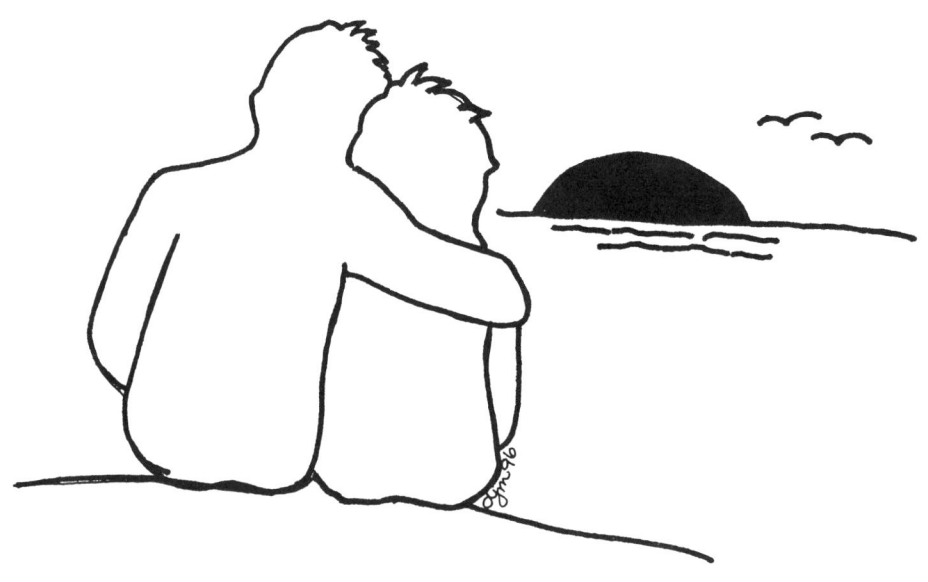

Peaceful Spirit
Terry Gonsoulin

Especially at night
It gets lonely
Too much time to think
Thoughts, fears, panic
Swirl around in my head
But
Slowly a spirit envelopes me
The peaceful spirit speaks ever so softly
I'm here
to keep you safe
to love you
to heal you

Terry Gonsoulin, age 39, of Oklahoma City. Terry is a registered nurse and serves as administrative director of the Troy & Dollie Smith Cancer Center at INTEGRIS Baptist Medical Center in Oklahoma City. Terry, diagnosed at age 31, is also a wife and mother. She is active in several cancer-related organizations, and is Chair of Project Woman, a committee of the Oklahoma Division of the American Cancer Society which educates women about breast cancer.

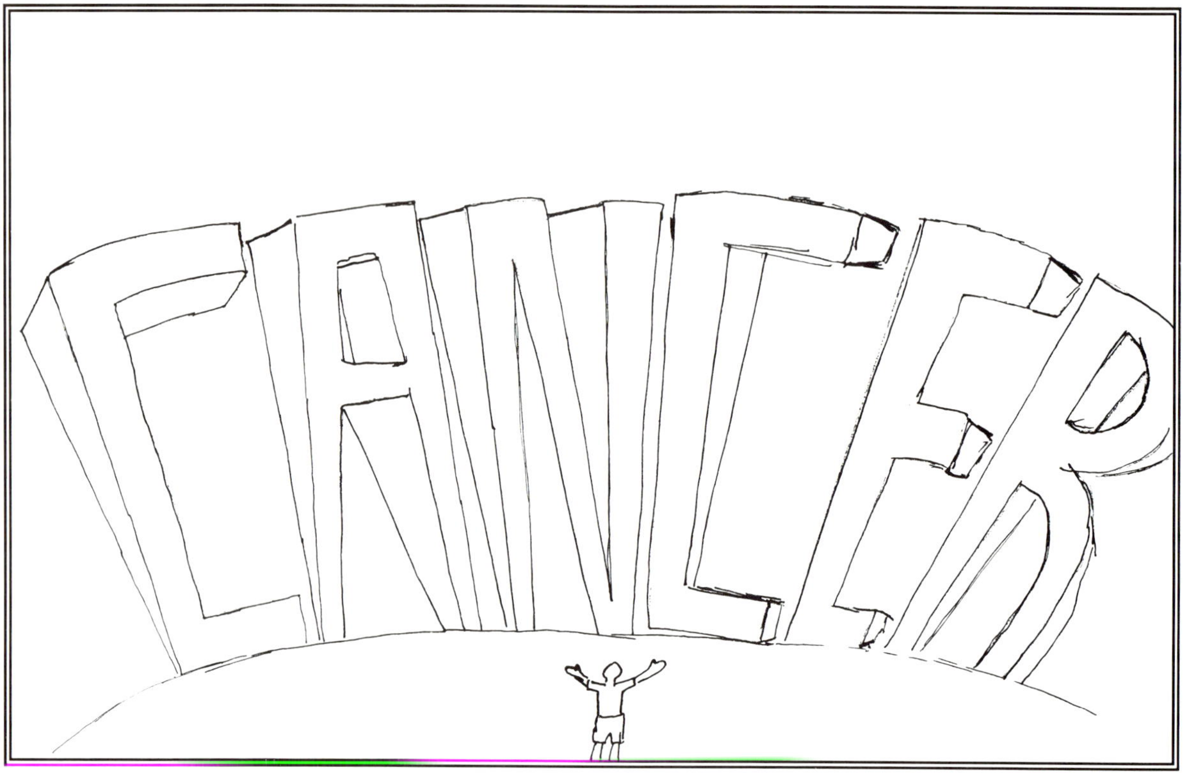

"A Child's Point of View"

Andrew Chandler (age 16)
Addison Chandler (age 9)

Through the Eyes of a Child
Dena Drabek

Regardless of your age, the news of cancer always comes as a shock. And along with the diagnosis comes disbelief, anger, fear, guilt, depression, grief, and heartache. It is hard to believe that anything like this could happen to someone you know and love so much. As seen through the eyes of a child, everything changes. It's like a bomb has been dropped! They live in a world of hurt, not knowing what to expect. They are headed for an emotional rollercoaster. Some children are full of questions right from the start. Is it contagious? Am I going to get it? Are you going to die? For others, it doesn't hit until later; then, after it has begun to set in, they start to think about what could happen. Still other kids seem to have nerves of steel and refuse to show any emotion at all; they just shut it out, so to speak. Each individual response varies according to the child's temperament, background, emotional and physical health, and age.

As if it's not hard enough to cope with the emotions at home, things can be even harder at school. Relationships with friends don't always turn out the way you expect them to. Some become closer friends and stand by you through the good times and the bad—sympathetic to you. Others are cruel and turn their backs. Teachers also play a role in this. It is usually best to inform your teachers of what's going on at home. This will prepare them for problems that may affect your school work in the future. It also helps them to be more sensitive and understanding of your needs, especially when it comes time for surgeries and treatments.

This is usually the toughest time for most kids. The terms lumpectomy, mastectomy, radiation, and Kemotherapy* usually don't register in a child's vocabulary—making the whole experience even harder to understand. Komen Kids™, Kids Helping Kids has been able to help children with this by letting them know that they are not alone. Art therapists and oncologist nurses come to answer questions and talk with kids on their level. Kids also get to see what cancer looks like.

This gives kids more understanding as to what is going on—something that they can grasp and actually hold on to. Many of them say that Komen Kids™ has made them more knowledgeable about cancer and the effect it has on everyone. Now, when they see other kids affected by cancer, they aren't afraid to reach out to them in a way that they would not have known before.

The following stories are true first-hand experiences based on Dena's interviews with children who are members of Komen Kids™, a program of the Central Oklahoma Chapter of the Susan G. Komen Breast Cancer Foundation.

Dena Drabek, age 15, of Moore. Dena is a member of Komen Kids™, a support group for children of loved ones facing life-threatening illnesses. Dena has composed this preface and the following brief stories of children's experiences as they see their mothers confront breast cancer.

*Dena and the other Komen Kids™ know how to spell chemotherapy. They have adopted a new, short-hand spelling (Kemo) of this word which has come to be all too familiar to their lives and vocabularies.

The Goetts

November of 1991, Elizabeth Goett was informed that her mother, Cathy, had fallen victim to breast cancer. This for a young elementary child was a lot to take in. Elizabeth, the oldest of two children, had many questions; the first being, "Is it contagious?" Her brother, then too young to understand, pretty much stayed out of harm's way. Elizabeth now considers herself very fortunate that her mother's situation was not as bad as some of the other members of Komen Kids™. Her mother not having to go through the radiation and Kemotherapy that is usually necessary, made it easier on them. Now leading a healthy cancer-free life, Cathy Goett is coming upon her six-year anniversary of remission.

Interviewed by Dena Drabek.

The Hepners

The Hepners' story is a little different simply because Tifani's mother, Sue, has not recovered and is still undergoing treatments and surgeries. It all started in August of 1993 when she was diagnosed. Since then she has had a masectomy, bone marrow transplant, Kemotherapy, and radiation therapy. Tifani has found for her the best way to get through this is one day at a time. She has learned from sessions of Komen Kids™ that it is good to talk things out and share your feelings. The hardest part for her has been watching her mom go through all the Kemo and radiation. But her dad, Bill, is always there for her when she needs him. Her advice to anyone in the same situation is just take it day by day and hang in there. It has worked for her.

Interviewed by Dena Drabek.

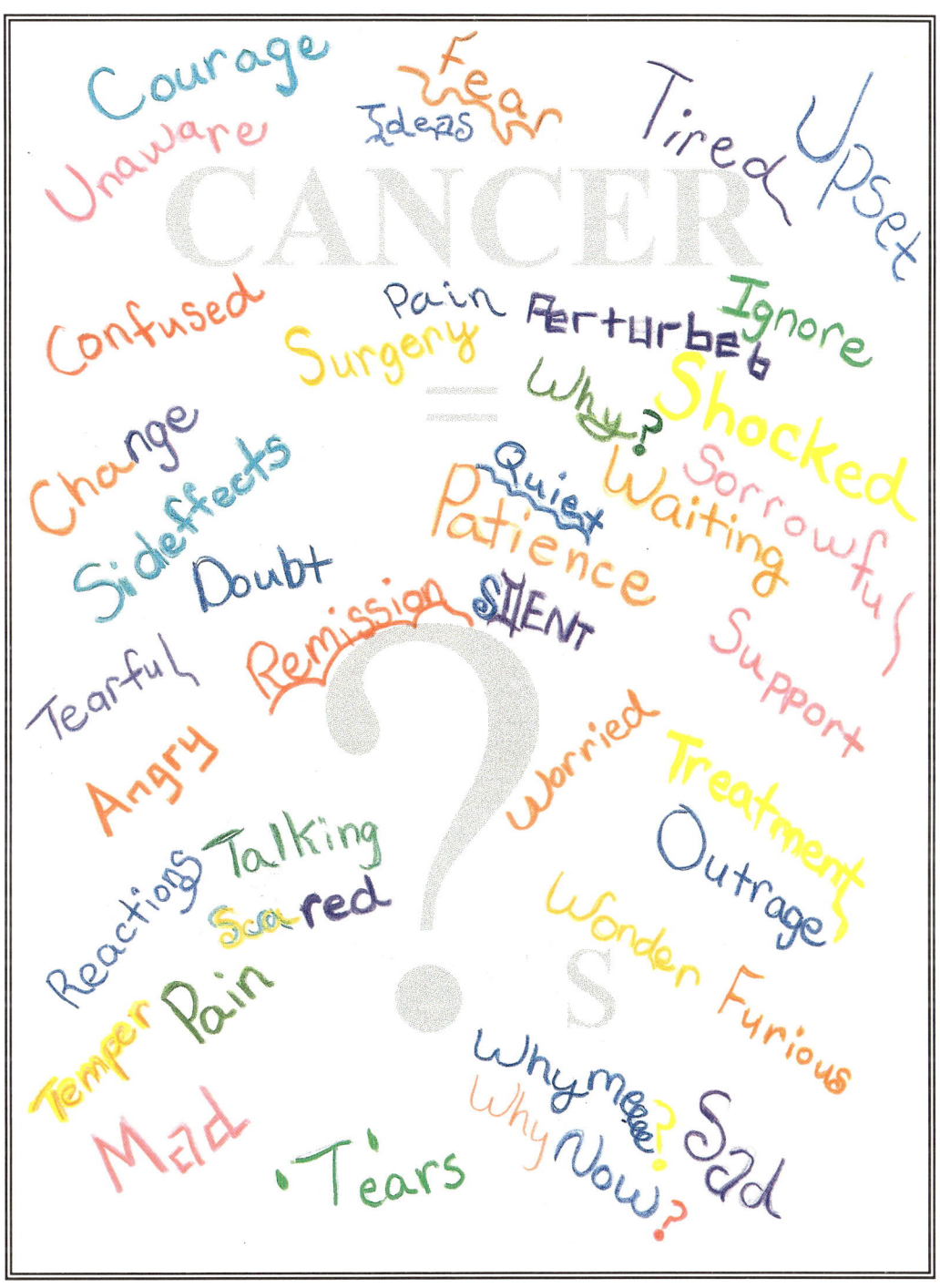

"There Are So Many Questions"   Elizabeth Goett (age 13)

The Bells

It has been three years since Tony's mother was diagnosed with breast cancer.* To this day she is still fighting and is determined to recover. She has been through two mastectomies, lung surgery, Kemotherapy, and radiation therapy. Tony is now 10 and tries not to think about his mother's diagnosis. He has learned to shut it out. He doesn't like to show his emotions and gets through most of it on his own. When he does want to know about something, he usually reads up on it or he talks to his dad. Tony does admit that he does have hard times. His hardest times are probably seeing his mother through all the surgeries she has been through.

Tony's mother, Bernadette Margaret McGowan Bell, died May 24, 1996.
Interviewed by Dena Drabek.

The Chandlers

Andrew and Addison, now ages 16 and 9, are recovering from the pain and torment their family endured during their mother's diagnosis of breast cancer throughout the year of 1994. Connie's treatments and surgeries included a mastectomy, Kemotherapy, and reconstruction surgeries. During that year, Andrew and Addison both did a lot of growing up. They relied on Komen Kids to help them understand what their mom was going through and how to deal with their emotions and fears. Andrew, President of the Oklahoma Chapter of Komen Kids, Kids Helping Kids, says that it has helped him and his brother to share their feelings with other kids. The Chandlers have comfort in knowing that Connie's cancer is now in remission.

Interviewed by Dena Drabek.

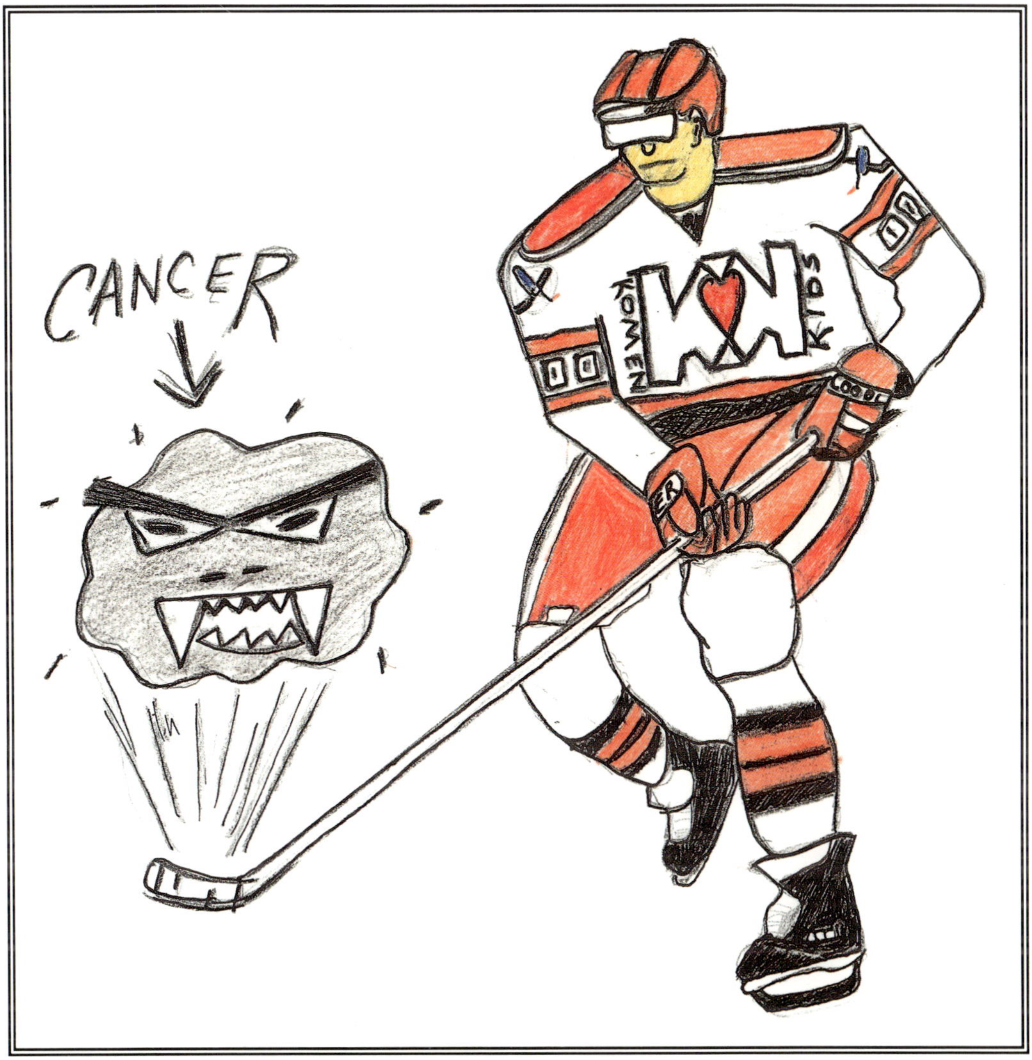

"The Hockey Player"   Andrew Chandler (age 16)

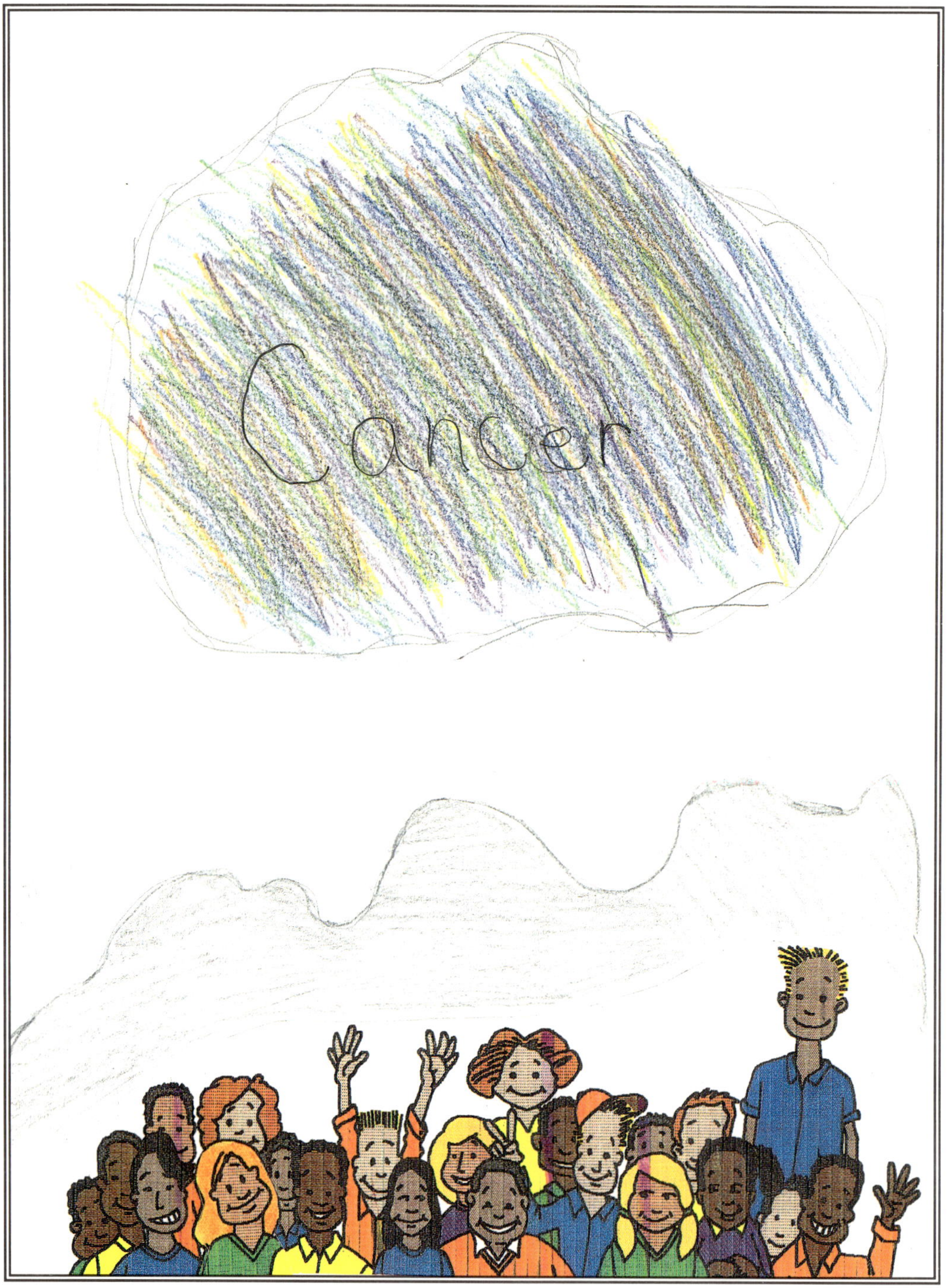

"The Cloud of Cancer
Shadows Your Life"

Elizabeth Goett (age 13)

You Are Not Alone
Komen Kids

~⌒

When you feel like no one's there,
and your family needs your care,
but the burden is so great for such a young child

There is a place to go,
where the sorrow is but hope,
where kids are helping kids to make it through.

You are not alone,
we are there to get you through.
The pain is eased by the sharing and the caring.

Komen Kids is our support
for feelings out of sort.
Joining hands across the way and knowing we are not alone.

You are not alone.
I am not alone.
We are not alone.

~⌒

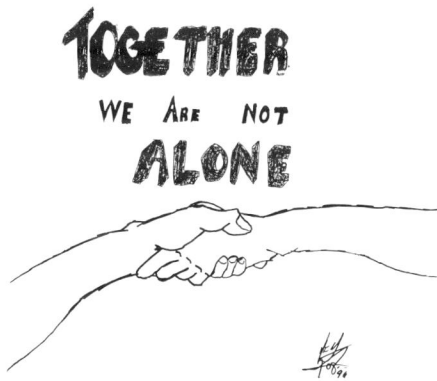

This theme song was composed by children in Komen Kids, a program of the Central Oklahoma Chapter of the Susan G. Komen Breast Cancer Foundation. The line art, entitled "Together We Are Not Alone," was drawn by Nick Mosley, age 13.

7
A New Outlook on Life
"Some things are not as important."

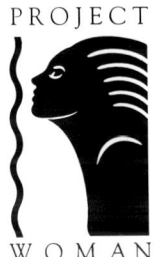

7

A New Outlook on Life

"Some things are not as important."

⁓

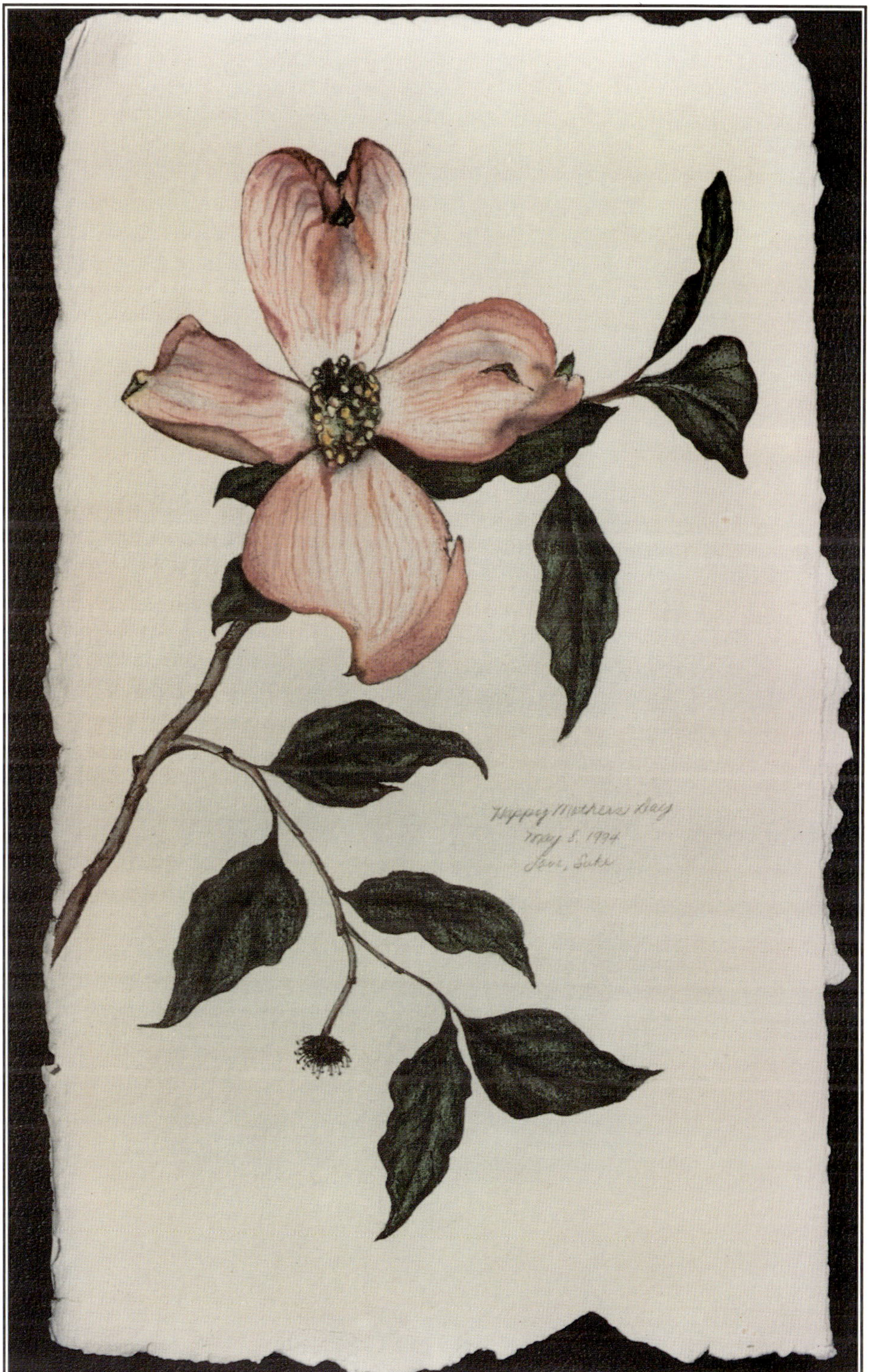

"Mom's Dogwood"   Jacque Collins Young

Jacque indicates that she did this painting for her mother as a Mother's Day gift.

Some Things Are Not as Important
Fern Peery

I had a modified radical mastectomy, followed by radiation. A Reach to Recovery visitor came to me while I was still in the hospital, offering an assortment of printed information, a hand exerciser, and prosthesis. As soon as I was able to go out socially again, my husband and I got involved in a cancer support group. I read about an "I Can Cope" course and went to every meeting by myself. I teamed up with a woman from a nearby town, and we enjoyed visiting at the meetings. I saved hand-outs when she missed meetings. I was surprised to read her obituary. Another participant who was so dear to all of us also died. That hits hard. But we were all in there trying to do our best to live each day to the fullest. We all tried to hold each other up. We cared. We looked at the present and the future realistically.

I think about this often. I have successfully passed the first-year anniversary of my survival. I have worked on my priorities. I realize some things are not as important as I had always thought. I look at relationships I hope to enrich. I believe this:

> When you have come to the edge of all the light you know,
> And are about to step off into the darkness of the unknown,
> Faith is knowing one of two things will happen:
> There will be something solid to stand on,
> Or you will be taught how to fly.
>
> *—author unknown*

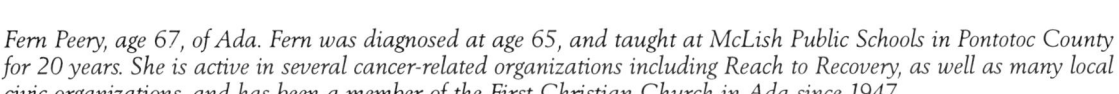

Fern Peery, age 67, of Ada. Fern was diagnosed at age 65, and taught at McLish Public Schools in Pontotoc County for 20 years. She is active in several cancer-related organizations including Reach to Recovery, as well as many local civic organizations, and has been a member of the First Christian Church in Ada since 1947.

Reaching for the Stars
Eleanor Yturria Irvin

The first thing the doctor said was that there had been a bad report from the mammogram and that I needed to be in the surgeon's office the next day. I went to his office and we both looked at the mammogram. He stated that he believed there was cancer and I would need to go into the hospital the following week for a biopsy. When I awoke from the surgery, I immediately asked my mother the results of the biopsy. She tried to hide being upset. I then turned to my friend Carol. Her response was that most feared answer, "You have cancer." So in my distress I went to the Lord in prayer. I knew He would provide restoration and the perfect help I needed. There were so many miracles during that time. As I walked into the clinic to find out about the chemotherapy, I saw a rainbow in the sky and Carol said that was my promise from God that all would be well. Since that time I have been greatly blessed even in adversity.

In June of 1995, I went to the Cancer Center in Arlington, Texas, for my annual checkup. I had felt a lump in the breast where I had the lumpectomy but did not mention it to my doctor. I figured that my tests were good and, after all, I had a biopsy in the summer of '94 and it was only scar tissue. This was most likely the same thing. Yet, I felt some urgency to call the doctor. The week before I went to the surgeon, I felt really tired and confessed to myself that it felt much like before when I had cancer. When the doctor examined me this time, he said I needed a biopsy right away. Two days later, I flew to Arlington for a scintigram. After administering the test, the radiologist came to me in the hallway and informed me that he was afraid a malignant tumor had shown up. My feeling was that of disbelief. It was as if the doctor was talking to someone else, not me. In spite of it, a calm came over me and I began singing to myself, "Nearer My God to Thee."

A mammogram and sonogram confirmed the scintigram reading. Upon seeing the reports, the doctor informed me that my only suitable options were a mastectomy and chemotherapy. On November 9th I went for the surgery. Again, I felt the Lord's presence and knew that He was in control. The next three weeks were filled with praying, trusting God and believing Him for a good pathology report. In December, the doctor reviewed my pathology report and, to my relief, announced that I was a candidate for tamoxifen instead of chemotherapy. It is hard to hold back the tears and realize that the Lord and I have this battle again. But, I continue to reach out to help other women with breast cancer, and I continue reaching for the stars and all the promises and blessings the Lord has for my life.

Eleanor Yturria Irvin, age 46, of Tulsa. Eleanor, initially diagnosed at age 41, is an art teacher, painter, and children's book author. She has been actively involved in several cancer-related organizations, and started a support group that meets monthly for dinner and discussion.

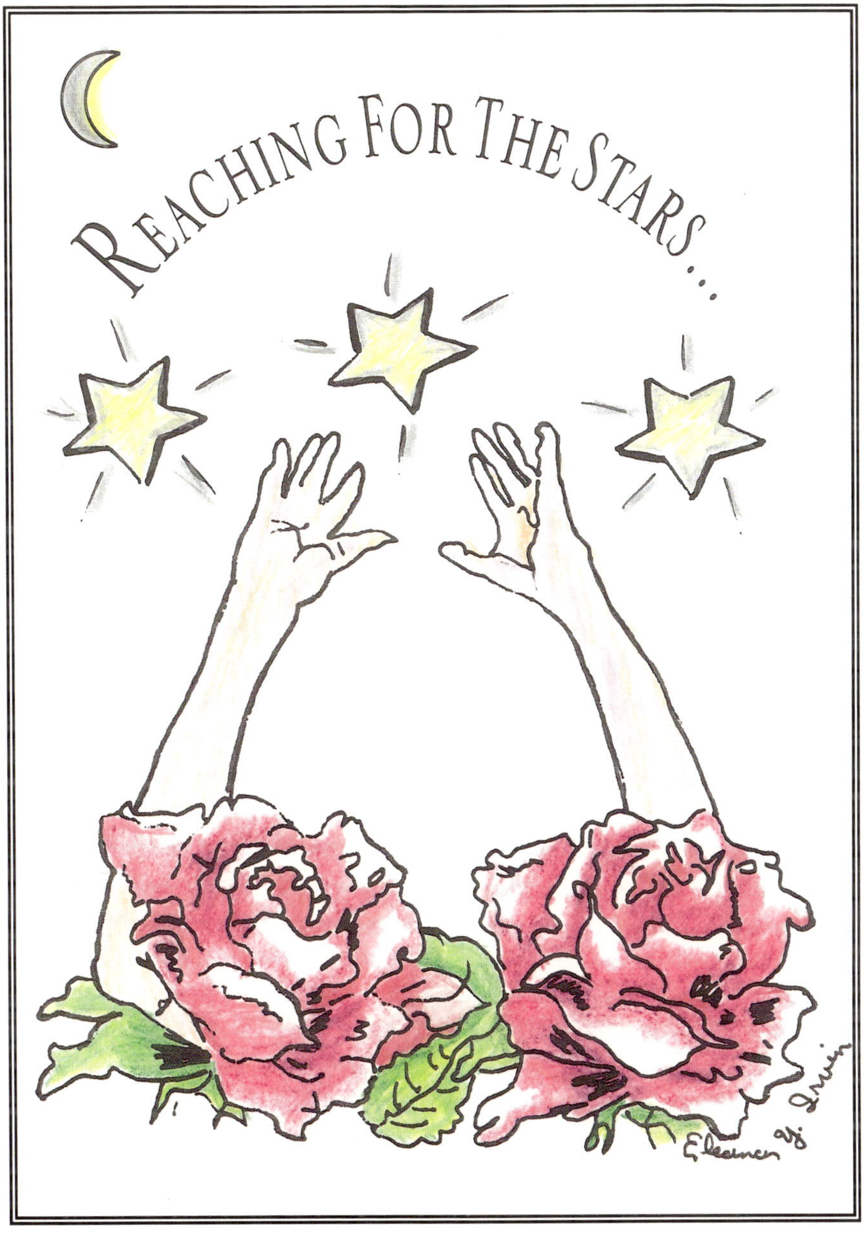

"Reaching for the Stars"   Eleanor Yturria Irvin

More Precious Now
Cherlyn Wilferth

It has been two years since I heard those scary words: breast cancer. But I've found there is life after surgery, chemotherapy, and radiation. I am so grateful the cancer was detected at the stage it was. A lot of new research is happening for breast cancer, but it is up to us to spread the word about self-exams, mammograms, and early detection. Life was great before. It is ever more precious now.

Cherlyn Wilferth, age 48, of Woodward. Cherlyn, a hairdresser in Woodward for 20 years, was first diagnosed at age 46. She is a single working mother of two and grandmother of three who has handled her work, parenting, and her cancer treatments very well. She provides wigs to cancer patients, as well as hair styling and cuts to chemotherapy patients.

No Longer Afraid
Linda Parker

My life now is filled with many new friends that I've made since my mastectomy and bone marrow transplant. My relationships with my grown children are better than ever and I'm married to a wonderful, supportive husband. I've found a hobby that I dearly love, doing stained glass. I've never been creative and was afraid to try, but now I'm no longer afraid.

Life is precious and you have to fight for it! Each day is a new beginning, and we can waste it or use it for good. My advice: find something you enjoy doing and do a lot of it. Keep a good attitude and give back what you can to help others. Be gentle with yourself and cultivate your inner spiritual awareness.

Linda Parker, age 54, of Edmond. For most of her adult life, Linda has been employed as either a bookkeeper or a secretary, but for the past eight years she has been a sales assistant for a major brokerage house. She was diagnosed at age 50, and has been involved in several cancer-related organizations including Reach to Recovery, Camp Live-A-Dream, and serves as an on-call volunteer at Oklahoma Memorial Hospital to talk with people who are preparing for a bone marrow transplant.

Looks for the Good
Betty Jane Bergman

Betty represents life's struggle with breast cancer. Always a picture of health, she breast-fed three children, never smoked or drank, and she believes that God is her strength. Her faith was tested in March 1978. She continued to teach, however, while taking 25 radiation treatments and a year of chemotherapy. This was a real challenge for her since she had been "mutilated" (this was her word for quite some time); and she could not understand how or why this would happen to her. But she has given strength to many of her friends in overcoming and coping with new health problems. She always looks for the good and finds it. She says that her bout with cancer made her appreciate what great blessings she has.

Betty Jane Bergman, age 66, of Pryor. Submitted by her daughter, Lisa Dennis. Betty was diagnosed at age 49, and has been a public school teacher for 30 years. She feels her years of teaching, and her husband, children, grandchildren, friends, reading, and gardening have made for a very rich and stimulating life. She is active in the Reach to Recovery program, as well as the First Baptist Church and several educators' organizations.

A Job to Be Done
Franke Rayburn

I accepted the presidency of the Pittsburg County Unit of the American Cancer Society in 1983, not because I had a close relationship with a cancer patient but because it was a job to be done. I had been a member of the Board for three years. Little did I know that I would be diagnosed with breast cancer in 1986. After two mastectomies and a rapid recovery, I realized what the American Cancer Society can mean to a cancer patient.

This experience has helped me to focus on the really important things in life—to appreciate God's gifts to me: a wonderful husband, two great children, a fine son-in-law, two super grandsons, a granddaughter-in-law and now an adorable great-granddaughter. Why should I complain? I've had a wonderful life.

Franke Rayburn, age 73, of McAlester. Franke, a homemaker, mother and "professional volunteer," was diagnosed at age 64. She has served as chair of the Pittsburg County American Cancer Society and other cancer-related organizations, and is the organist for All Saints Episcopal Church. She is active in Rain Team, an AIDS support organization, and she tutors for the Literacy Council.

In This Past Year
Roseanna D. Smith

In this past year...
I have never been so close to death
  and I have never felt so alive.
I have never been so ill
  nor have I ever experienced such radiant health.

I have never been so fearful and anxious
  yet never have I felt such tranquillity and peace.
Never have I felt such distance from God,
  and never have I felt so close and connected.

Never have I been so loved
  nor have I loved so deeply.
I have never felt so lost and searching
  yet as close to understanding the meaning and purpose of life.

I have read more books within this past year
  than in all the years preceding.
I have told physicians what I will do and what I will not do.
  I have even told physicians how they can improve their communication
  with other patients.

I have eliminated people and experiences from my life
  which I felt were not conducive to my health.
And I have surrounded myself with people
  who can be my teachers and nurturers.

I have reduced the crap from my life
  and replaced it with experiences
Which I enjoy
  and which provide me my greatest learning.

In this past year...

I have added new words to my language:
  white blood count... 5-FU...
Prednisone... proliferate... prognosis...
  LaShan... Bernie Siegel... hypnotherapy

Now I stop to smell the roses.
  I gaze at sunsets.
I even look at individual blades of grass
  and individual leaves on trees.

I see so much more clearly
  the way the hair grows on my husband's head,
The way he grins when he thinks he is in trouble
  and the glorious way he laughs when he experiences joy.

In this past year...

I lost friends who were too afraid
  to face their own mortality.
 And yet, I experienced friendship so beautiful
  that it still remains indescribable.

I was exhausted by the chemicals.
  I was invigorated by the challenge.
I came from a place of fear and aloneness
  and gained a mission of sharing and hope.

Roseanna D. Smith, age 53, of Oklahoma City, was diagnosed in 1990 at age 49. She is a Licensed Marriage and Family Therapist and a breast cancer survivor. Roseanna facilitates cancer support groups and devotes a significant portion of her time to those who face life threatening illnesses. She is an active volunteer for the American Cancer Society and serves as Chair of the Book Committee responsible for producing this publication as Phase II of Project Woman, A Portrait of Breast Cancer: Expressions in Words and Art.

The Best Is Yet to Come
Kathy Jane Perkins

Like a whirlwind, Kathy was always busy, effervescent, upbeat, with a smile that made you know her hands and heart went out to everyone whose life she touched. But, cancer is no respecter of persons or age. In 1988, at age 30, Kathy was first diagnosed with breast cancer. Four years later, she surrendered her fragile hold on life with rare dignity and grace.

Shortly before her death, Kathy consented to an interview with a local staff writer, Jackie Holston. The following are excerpts of that interview.

In April 1988, Kathy, believing she was pregnant, went to a Tulsa physician for a checkup. During that examination a lump was discovered in her breast. The doctor told her she was too young to have cancer, nothing to worry about. Reassured, she went home and did become pregnant a few months later. She had also been examined by one other doctor who told her she need not be concerned. "Then," she said, "I went to another doctor who discovered that a tumor in my breast was cancerous. It had grown from the size of a pea to the size of a lemon." To halt the cancer's growth, her pregnancy was terminated and she underwent a hysterectomy and mastectomy.

Angry at the doctors and momentarily questioning God, Kathy wondered if things might have been different had something been done sooner. She believed it is important for people to question their physician if they do not feel comfortable about a diagnosis, and to seek several different opinions if necessary. By telling her story she hoped to save someone else the pain her family had to experience.

Kathy believed her illness gave her a new perspective on life. "Small things like the sound of falling rain or the fragrance of flowers were greatly savored." She learned to set things aside and spend time with the people who meant the most to her. "Things will wait," she said. And in conclusion, Kathy reflected, "I have come to realize that you live your life on earth and the best is yet to come."

Kathy Jane Perkins, of Pryor, died at age 34. This story was submitted in her memory by her mother-in-law, Beverly Perkins, including excerpts from an interview by Jackie Holston, Staff Writer, The Daily Times, Pryor, Oklahoma. Kathy was initially diagnosed at age 30. A wife and mother, Kathy had been a checker at the Homeland grocery store, was active in church activities at Bethlehem Lutheran Church, as well as Little League, PTA, and the Pryor chapter cancer support group.

Each Day Is a Gift
Judy McGee

Each day is a gift from the Lord,
treasure it;
Don't take it for granted;
live it to the fullest, use it wisely.
Find time to laugh, to love, to listen, to care.
Find time to be alone with God.
Choose to be happy and
to help others find happiness.
If we can achieve these things
we will find true joy and peace in life.

Judy McGee, age 48, of Oklahoma City. Judy was diagnosed at age 44, and is an artist and homemaker. Her faith in God has helped her in the fight against breast cancer.

8
Giving Something Back
"They believe you when you've been there."

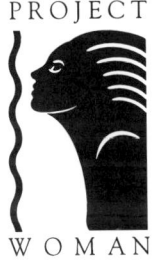

8
Giving Something Back
"They believe you when you've been there."

～つ

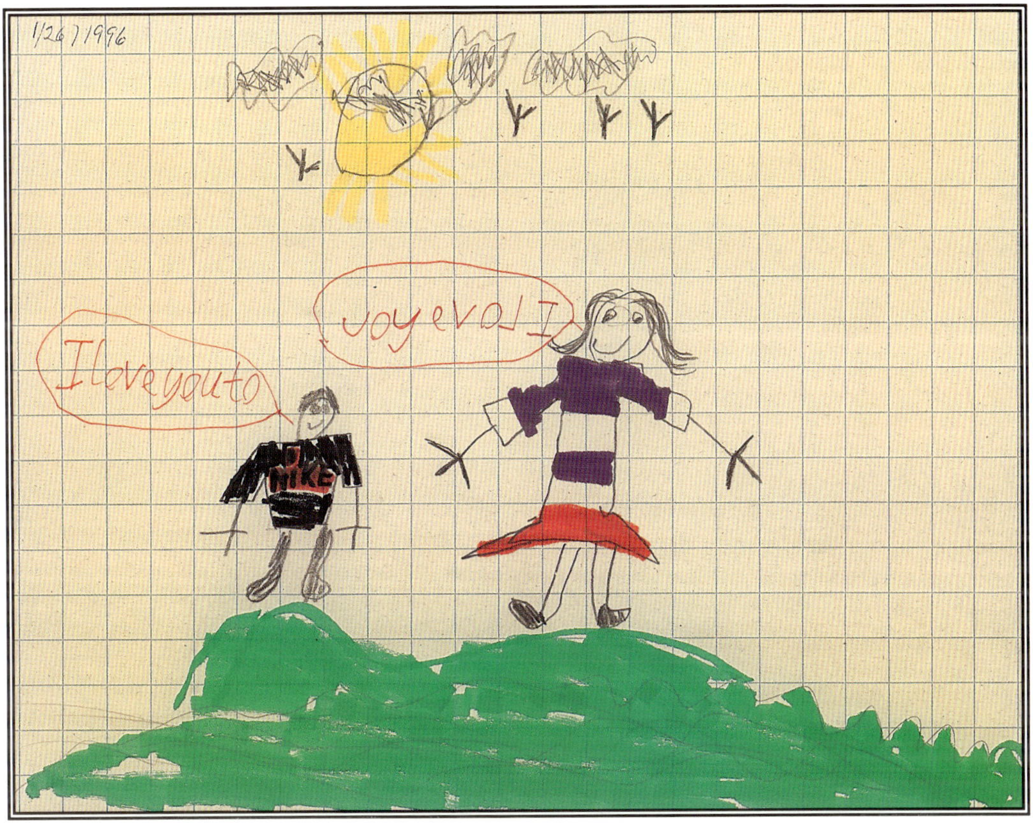

"Mom Will Keep Watching Over Me"   **Christopher Gilbert**

This is a drawing by Christopher Gilbert, age 8, of himself and his mother, Dr. Kerri Williams. According to Christopher's grandmother, Lonnie Williams, "He did this painting 17 days after his Mom's death. He is talking to his Mom and she is talking to him. That's why the words are reversed." Kerri Williams' story is on pages 146-147.

They Believe You When You've Been There
Becky Loveall

It could have been a life-changing trauma; instead Becky turned it into an opportunity to give to others who faced the uncertainties of breast cancer. She had a modified radical mastectomy and, because of lymph node involvement, it was followed by chemotherapy and radiation. She uses her position in the radiology department at Tulsa Regional Medical Center as a chance to counsel the patients she meets, and she represents the hospital at health fairs where she enjoys the one-on-one contacts she makes. "People tend to believe you if you have already had the experience," Becky believes. "I feel they walk away feeling better about treatment. I enjoy talking someone through their apprehensions." After reconstructive surgery, she volunteered to be a resource person for her plastic surgeon and she talks with women who are contemplating this avenue.

At first it was hard for Becky, especially losing her hair and wearing a wig to work. She remembers the night of the Catoosa tornado in 1993, when hospital staff was called in. Her wig had just been washed and she had to report in without it, in her own very short hair. But her co-workers gave her so many positive comments, she never looked back again.

And, her philosophy of life has changed. "Nothing in life is so great to get upset about," she believes. Now she faces life with a calmer, more laid back attitude.

Becky Loveall, age 41, of Tulsa. Submitted by her friend, Jerry Jones. Becky was diagnosed at age 37, and works as a radiology scrub technician. In her career, she enjoys talking with patients about their fears of breast cancer, as she feels it relaxes them to know they can get through it. She is an active volunteer for the American Cancer Society, represents her employer at health fairs and charity drives, participates in her son's hockey league organizations, and is a volunteer counselor to cancer patients.

No Time for a Mammogram
Norma Codding

I felt that my schedule was just too busy to take time for a mammogram. That was for those other people. I did not give my own body special attention. I felt I must go and give my time to others. I even volunteered at the hospital to schedule other women for mammograms. And when I finally did schedule myself, I gave my first and second appointment times to someone else. But because of the loving support of my volunteer friends, they called me for that unscheduled mammogram.

To my surprise, the diagnosis was breast cancer. A biopsy and a modified radical mastectomy followed within the week. Joy has replaced surprise and anger; I'm thankful to be a survivor. The support of friends and family have replaced feelings of abandonment; they scheduled that appointment and then stood by me to this day.

My experience of breast cancer has broadened my life with new understanding and direction. I visit breast cancer patients through the Reach to Recovery program. I propose to share my experience with this admonition: take special care of and give time to thyself, be positive and have fierce determination to live life in spite of it all.

I have received various honors and awards by serving individuals, families and the community through volunteer service. But one of my greatest feelings slipped up on me—the evening that I participated in the survivor's "Relay for Life," a team event to fight cancer— I walked and wore my T-shirt proudly!

Norma Codding, age 65, of Stillwater. Norma was diagnosed at age 60, and has been a school teacher and community volunteer for several years. She has worked on committees for virtually every health concern in existence, including AIDS, organ/tissue donor awareness, cancer, Special Olympics, traffic safety, infant mortality, drug prevention and abuse and others. She was named one of five volunteers of the year at the annual "Five Who Care" awards sponsored by KOCO-TV in Oklahoma City, and received a City of Stillwater proclamation declaring "Norma Codding Day" in honor of her community service to that city.

Ease Their Fears
Rhota J. Chapman

Rhota's life isn't much different from yours, mine or most women's. She has been a loving wife to Sonny for 39 years, is a mother of three children and a grandmother of seven grandchildren. But, in 1988, Rhota noticed a sore spot on her breast. She was diagnosed with breast cancer and a modified radical mastectomy was performed.

Because of Rhota's strong desire to help others, she went to school to become an LPN and after ten years of nursing and further education, she became an RN. During her 16 years at the hospital, Rhota has affected many lives. She is a confident and caring nurse. It is especially wonderful for the mastectomy patients whom Rhota asks to care for. In addition to their physical needs, she often sits beside her patients and talks with them to ease their fears. She shares her own experiences of breast cancer and has even shown her physical scar to those who are curious as to how the breast heals. "There are much worse things in life than breast cancer," are words of encouragement she offers to friends, patients, and coworkers.

Rhota Chapman, age 57, of Midwest City. Submitted by her friends and coworkers: Sherry Cooper, Myra Henry, Mandy Ober, and Debbie Whiting. A registered nurse at Midwest City Regional Hospital, Rhota has spent her life dedicated to helping others. She was diagnosed at age 49.

This Happened for a Purpose
Teddy McMillon

My mom is the neatest person I know. She represents the "winning spirit" of breast cancer. Her mission is to help others through the crisis that she also experienced. Teddy comes by her talents naturally, following in the footsteps of her parents, Ted and Bertha Fruechting, who also had cancer and spent their lives in service to others.

Teddy travels across the state of Oklahoma as a representative of the American Cancer Society and as a Reach to Recovery lady. Her lighthearted approach to discussing this serious subject has allowed her to reach women of all ages, such as talking to a high school home economics class about self-breast examinations or encouraging senior citizens not to forget that it's never too late to get your first mammogram.

While she has worked with the American Cancer Society (current state board member) since 1987 when her father died, she did not, as she puts it, "become impassioned with cancer until I became a 'one boob lady' in 1991." When this occurred, she adds, "I felt this happened for a purpose and I wanted to share my experience with others."

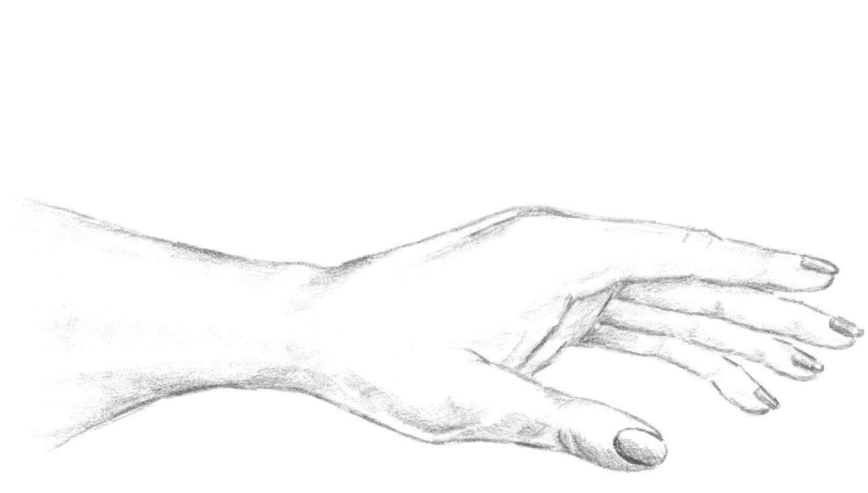

Teddy McMillon, age 61, of Weatherford. Submitted by her daughters, Donise Woods and Kimberly McMillon. Teddy was an army wife for 23 years, and is a mother of three children and grandmother of seven. A "professional volunteer," Teddy is involved in several major civic and health organizations. She presents humorous and entertaining programs on breast cancer awareness and the importance of early detection to women's groups of all ages. She was diagnosed at age 57.

Why Me?
Frances Louise Fisher

It was malignant, a carcinoma and very aggressive. Upon leaving the doctor's office I kept asking myself, "Why me?" That night I called a woman from our church, Judy. She had been through this tormenting experience only six months before and had just finished her chemotherapy. She immediately came to my house and counseled me as to what to expect. It was reassuring. Judy was my Godsend.

The following day I had a modified mastectomy of the right breast. Then came the weeks of recovery. As soon as possible I anxiously returned to work teaching my third graders. That is where I needed to be. I had to get my mind off that inner voice saying, "Why me?"

Chemotherapy definitely was no "treat" but I knew it was the way to treat my cancer. Shortly after the first chemo treatment, I lost my hair. I was bald! Again, "Why me?"

Three and half years later, I realize how vulnerable we are. It can happen to any one of us. But I no longer dwell on "Why me?". God left me here for a purpose. Now I ask, "What can I do for others like me?" I intend to fulfill that purpose. I know I can make a difference in someone else's life as Judy did in mine.

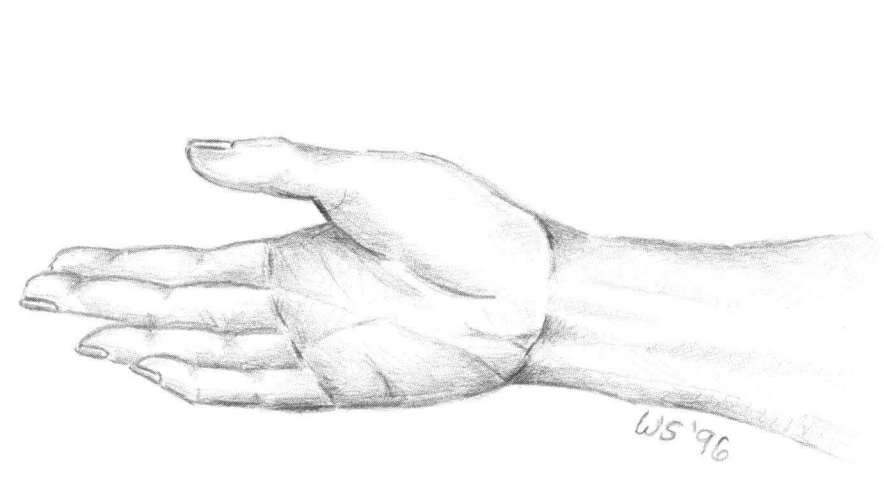

Frances "Louise" Fisher, age 47, of Woodward. Louise, who earned both bachelor's and master's degrees in education, has taught elementary school in Woodward for 25 years. She is a lector, eucharistic minister, cantor, and minister to the homebound for her church. A wife, mother, and grandmother as well, she was diagnosed at age 43.

A Small Part in Helping
Grace F. Hollrah

My father and I were born on the same farm that my grandfather staked at the Oklahoma Land Run. In 1941, I married Roy and we raised four boys. We are now enjoying the fruits of our 55+ years of marriage at the "old homestead." But in 1973, having just been informed that I had breast cancer, and no other family member had had this disease, I was devastated. The trauma for me was real. First we question why, then tears come, but God has a way of helping us by giving us time. This lessens the tears and fears and we begin to get on with our lives, and helping others. I lost my breast but had all my other faculties.

My life has since been devoted to community service and volunteer work. My first love is my cancer work. I first volunteered for the Reach to Recovery program, and have been doing it now for 21 years. I have no idea how many Reach to Recovery visits I've made. Then I had the urge to do more, so I asked a nurse friend at the hospital if she thought a support group would work. Did it ever! (I remember for me there was no one to talk to or to give me a shoulder to lean on.) In eight years our support group has had over 2,500 people in attendance, representing 50 towns in northwest Oklahoma. We have given cancer talks, newspaper articles, testimonies, and programs of every kind that would help a person who has gone through this earth-shattering phase of their life. The thought remains with me that I had a small part in helping them cope with their lives.

But more, the quality of my own life has been better since my mastectomy. I found that I was a better person; many things that had been top priorities did not mean nearly as much after the operation. I did so much more for others and was rewarded in so many ways. For all of this, I pulled myself up by the bootstraps and gained a greater love of life.

Grace Hollrah, age 75, of Enid. Grace is a homemaker, a mother of four sons; she worked for several years in retail environments, as well as more than five years in senior citizen organizations. She was diagnosed at age 53. Grace embodies the strengths of her family heritage.

Hope Unlimited
Helen Kuhn

I was 83 in October, Breast Cancer Awareness month. Some 30 years ago, I had just completed the real estate and broker's tests. I was so pleased to pass them and was ready to go to work. But I knew something was wrong. I had been to the doctor at least a dozen times, at $4.00 per visit back then. Later that summer I had a radical mastectomy followed by cobalt. If only early detection had been stressed then, I might not have had to take cobalt.

I was the only volunteer in my area for Reach to Recovery (we called it Reach for Recovery) from 1970 to 1990. I could hardly wait to call on people. I wanted to talk to someone. I now belong to a support group named "Hope Unlimited." In October 1989, I was presented the Terese Lasser Award for outstanding service to the American Cancer Society, Oklahoma Division. Then, in 1995, I was surprised and so pleased to receive a plaque for "unselfish contribution to others for cancer research" from the American Cancer Society, Stephens County, Oklahoma Unit. The inscription quoted William James, "The best use of life is to spend it for something that outlasts life."

Helen Kuhn, age 83, of Duncan. She was diagnosed at age 53. She ran a successful real estate office until 1971. Helen has been a devoted volunteer for Reach to Recovery, serving in that role for the Duncan area from 1970 to 1990.

Great Inspiration
Beverly L. Mohr

Beverly was married for 35 years and was the mother of three children. She was fully devoted to her family. Those acquainted with her were impressed with how she could be so caring for others and yet not let her own pain and suffering be shown to them. She was a great inspiration to many other women who experienced cancer. Beverly was active in supporting cancer groups and cancer research. In fact, she participated in the UCLA/Revlon Research Program. As Beverly expressed it so compassionately, "If my participation in cancer research can help find a solution to this disease, then all the pain and suffering is worth it."

Beverly Mohr, of Tulsa, died at age 54. Submitted in her memory by her husband, Bill Mohr. Beverly, who was initially diagnosed at age 50, had been a revenue accountant for American Airlines. She was active in the "Y Me" cancer support group and other cancer-related organizations. She was also active in her church and loved her family and helped others to find quality and meaning in all aspects of their lives.

Can't Slow Down
Betty Dahms Lewis

～

This has not slowed me down or interfered with my work, travel, or remarriage at 71! I have worked for Reach to Recovery for 20 years. It is really great to visit with the patients and to see their attitude change from discouragement to hopefulness in 30 minutes or less. I tell them about when I had cancer and what I am doing. I review materials in the "kit" and answer their non-medical questions—exercise, everyday chores, dressing, where to find special garments—and the like. Often a husband or other interested adult will stay and listen and ask me questions, too.

～

Betty Dahms Lewis, age 75, of Stillwater. Betty was a teacher of home economics at Oklahoma State University for 30 years, and taught five years at the high school level. She was diagnosed at age 53, and has been an active Reach to Recovery volunteer for the past 20 years as well as volunteering for the American Red Cross. She is also an active church member, and recently remarried at the age of 71.

A Good Example
Beulah M. Attebery

～

Beulah found her breast tumor in 1965 after learning breast self-examination. She was treated with a modified radical mastectomy and cobalt and she lived 28 full years after the diagnosis. She was available to encourage cancer survival among other adult women. Long before it was popular, she increased women's knowledge about self care and physician follow-ups to find, treat, and prevent breast cancer. Beulah was a generous, courageous, and persistent woman who always sought the best for the other person, working to enhance the lives of other people. As she said, "If my life can ever benefit someone else's life, I hope I can always be a good example of life's joys."

～

Beulah Attebery, formerly of Tulsa, died at age 67. Submitted by her son and daughter-in-law, Bruce and Sandra Attebery. Beulah was diagnosed at age 39 after learning breast self-exam, and lived 28 years after her diagnosis. She was married more than 40 years, raised a son and daughter, was active in her church and enjoyed her three grandchildren.

Living and Loving Life
Bobbie Sue Wolf

Bobbie has invested her life in the lives of others, primarily her family. And she makes good sausage gravy, says Andy, her son-in-law. But she has contributed especially to the lives of women across Oklahoma who have discovered they are targets of cancer and are in need of a listening ear and words of encouragement. In a variety of volunteer services, Bobbie has been available to provide crucial support. Living and loving life is the legacy that Bobbie passes on to those near to her. As she has said, "Having cancer is not unique, but living with cancer with dignity and joy is."

Bobbie Sue Wolf, age 62, of Weatherford. Submitted by her daughters, Barbara Lou Deevers and Becky Sue Deck. Bobbie is a part-time clinic nurse volunteer, a homemaker and wife of an Air Force officer. She is a volunteer instructor for the Breast Self-Exam workshop at Clinton Hospital, and volunteers for numerous other community and church organizations.

Double Survivor
Jeane Yates

Jeane has been a model wife, mother, grandmother, teacher, and community leader in spite of her illness. Instead of focusing upon her own near tragedy, she has spent her energies in helping others through her extensive service to the American Cancer Society and more specifically through Reach Out visits. It should be noted that she is a double survivor in that she was first diagnosed with ovarian cancer in 1964 and then breast cancer in 1988. Her spirit is revealed in her statement, "Life is so precious! Yet, it is not the length that makes it so but, rather, the quality. We cannot always control what happens to us in this life, but we can control how we react. With a positive attitude and God by our side, we live each day to the fullest and inspire others."

Jeane Yates, age 69, of Stillwater. Submitted by her husband, Dr. Kyle Yates. Jeane was diagnosed at age 61, after first being diagnosed with ovarian cancer in 1964. She is acknowledged to be a model survivor in the face of her challenges.

You Never Know Whose Life You're Going to Touch
Kerri D. Williams

I was pregnant when I started my first year of residency, and had Christopher, my son, in December 1987. About four months later, I had quit breast feeding, and soon after felt a lump in my left breast while in the shower. While the mammogram was normal, there was something inside me that wasn't very easy with that, and I called my doctor. He said, "I want you in my office," and the next day we biopsied it, and it was malignant. I got out of the hospital from my first mastectomy two days before my 35th birthday. I underwent a modified radical mastectomy, and six months of chemotherapy, and then bilateral breast reconstruction with a prophylactic mastectomy on the right side.

I started my own practice in ophthalmology in 1991, and was doing quite well; then in October 1993, I felt a lump under my right arm, and it turned out to be a new primary breast cancer. It wasn't the same pathology as the first one, so I underwent six more months of chemotherapy. Then in May [1994] I developed a headache that just got progressively worse, to the point where I collapsed in the office one day on the bathroom floor. I called my doctor right away, and he said, "Get an MRI now." When we did that, it showed six or seven tumors in my brain and a large amount of cerebral edema, which was causing the headaches… I started radiation treatment, and the pressure came down. Subsequent CT scans showed tumors in the lung and liver. After additional treatments my latest scans showed my brain and liver to be completely clear, and my lung still has something in it… [The doctor] may present my case to the University for consideration for a stem cell transplant.

In some ways, I think Christopher twice helped save my life. The first time, when I was pregnant, the tumor grew, and if I hadn't been pregnant, that tumor might have sat there for many more years before it was detected. Christopher was also one of the main reasons I fought so hard this summer… Since he was now older, I felt we could go into more detail regarding my illness. We told him Mom was very sick, and that she had tumors in her head and body, and would have to take medical treatments to help fight them. Working as a family to deal with my illness might help him in the future to deal with other problems.

[B. Truels: *"Are we physicians so absorbed in our daily lives that we don't look beyond that?"*] It certainly gives you pause for reflection. I look at things very differently now. Life is very dear to me. That may sound kind of trivial, but you never know what's coming around the corner. I look at a lot of my friends, doctor-friends and otherwise, and I say, "Guys, life's too short, you're missing the message here." What's happened to me has made a lot of my friends more insightful as to where they're divvying up their time, and trying to make adjustments. If I'm able to help my friends in this way, then I know some good has come from all this.

The biggest thing I have learned… is that I have become a better doctor, because I've been through what a lot of my patients have been through. I have been through MRIs and CTs, bronchoscopies, and colonoscopies, and I've been poked and prodded and poisoned, and everything. It helps me understand what we do to our patients. And I don't think until you've walked in someone's shoes, you know what it's like. You touch people's lives in a different way. So many people were praying for me, and I truly believe that is what made those brain and liver tumors go away, along with the chemotherapy I'm taking—I don't discount the medicine, but I think that the miracle healing that I've experienced is very powerful. I don't think you can attribute it all to medicine… The physician needs help from other areas as well. Sometimes we make ourselves the judge and the jury as to how long we treat someone. More than once, I asked [my doctor] if it was time to give up. Each time, he told me, "No, but I will tell you when it is." That reassured me. That allowed me to reach down and find strength to fight. Patients want a true explanation, not a false hope. That's a fine line we have to walk as doctors.

I've told my story so long for the past seven years, but I think there's a purpose to it. It's a healing process for me. When they ask, I'm not hesitant to share it at all. It helps them too. You never know whose life you're going to touch, just by a simple comment or explanation, because they may be going through something similar that you don't even know about. We touch lives in a lot of different ways.

Kerri D. Williams, MD, of Oklahoma City, died in January 1996. Submitted in her memory by her husband, John Gilbert. Prior to her death, Dr. Williams was interviewed by William Truels, MD. The above story includes excerpts from that interview entitled, "Dealing with Adversity," as it appeared in the Oklahoma County Medical Society Bulletin. Kerry was an ophthalmologist with a thriving practice in Oklahoma City. She was married and had a small baby when she was first diagnosed, undergoing her first mastectomy two days before her 35th birthday. Active in her community, she was loved and admired by so many. In spite of her untimely death, Kerri's message of hope and optimism remains an inspiration to all. The artwork entitled "Mom Will Keep Watching Over Me" was drawn by Kerri's son, Christopher Gilbert, age 8. See page 135.

9
Paying Tribute
"She's my hero."

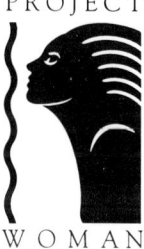

PROJECT
WOMAN

9
Paying Tribute
"She's my hero."

⟿

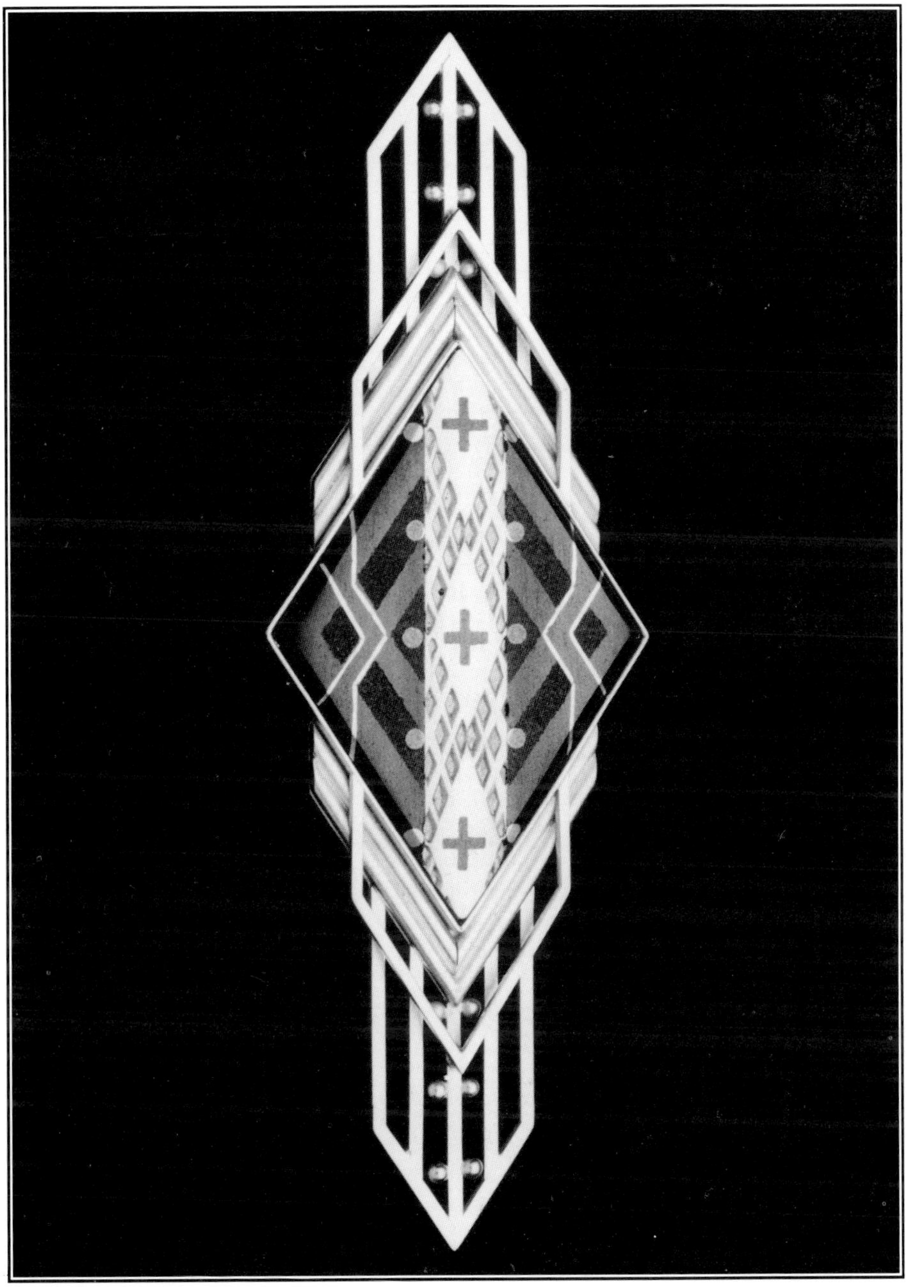

"New Mexico
Mourning Pin, #15"

Betsy Crump

This is a metal, enamel fabrication and enamel pin created by Betsy Crump in 1988. Photo by Sanford Mauldin.

She's My Hero
Missy Nobo

I am not a breast cancer survivor. I'm her sister. I was 34 when we found out Missy's tumor was malignant. The news came in a phone call from my mother. The rage that welled up in me was from the innermost depths. Rage at being a woman, at being in a high-risk group, and at my sister for letting this happen to her.

Afterall, she has always done everything right: straight A's, chaste until marriage, non-smoker, non-drinker, non-hedonist. She is beautiful and everyone has always respected her. Unfortunately, the cancer cells that invaded her body showed no respect. They didn't even have the decency to make themselves known. My sister was one of those whose mammogram showed no suspicious signs.

The chemo and radiation treatments were terrible, but she kept her humor and self-esteem intact. She even went back to work in the throes of nausea, teaching children with disabilities. She helped the kids to learn; they helped her to heal.

I'll share a secret with you: I made a deal with God. I promised him if he would make my sister well, I would give up everything—hopes for a marriage, having a child, financial success. No, I am not a martyr nor do I think it is against God's divine will. It was something I had to do.

Remember, we are talking about my sister, my friend, my mentor, my resident therapist. We are talking about the woman who took me shopping when I was so fat none of my clothes would fit; who sent me plane tickets to get me out of another mess; and who has always, unequivocally been there when I needed her.

We, my friends, are talking about my hero!

Submitted by Laurey Lummus, sister of Melissa (Missy) Nobo, age 45. Missy was diagnosed in June 1992, at age 41. She is a survivor and, just in case you didn't notice, she's Laurey's unabashed hero!

She Comforted Me
Patricia Ann Gordon

Wife, mother, grandmother, daughter, friend, and sister—my sister, Pat, was a generous spirit who took meals and communion to the home bound. Life was good; no signs of tragedy. Then in late 1984, her husband became seriously ill with pancreatic cancer. Pat quit work to care for him until his death in 1986.

Several months later Pat noticed a small lump in her breast. Within a year she endured a lumpectomy and radiation followed by a complete double mastectomy. She then met another man and was happily married. Her life was back on track and the family breathed a sigh of relief. But she developed a shoulder pain. It persisted and became worse. The x-ray showed bone cancer. By 1993, her cancer had spread to her skull, spine, legs, arms, lungs, liver and pancreas. The doctors estimated she had maybe four months to live. Nothing could be done but to keep her comfortable and to relieve her pain.

I refused to cry because I felt I had to be strong for her. One day, as I sat next to her bed thinking she was asleep, the tears came. I tried to be quiet so she would not hear, but she roused, reached over, patted my arm and said, "It will be alright." Here she was, knowing that she was dying, not crying for herself, and was still able to lend comfort to others.

That's who she was. She once said she was going to be in charge of her life and no matter what she faced in the time she had left, the cancer was not going to control her. She lived her life with strength and purpose. She died with dignity and grace. I am proud to call her my sister—and my friend.

Submitted by Glenda Schoen in memory of her sister, Patricia Ann Gordon, of Oklahoma City. Patricia died at the age of 55, following diagnosis at the age of 48. Her employment positions over the years ranged from secretary to office manager for an oral surgeon. After she quit work to care for her terminally ill husband and his subsequent death in 1986, she volunteered to help the homebound.

A Tribute
Jeane Malone

There's someone special I'd like you to meet;
Her name is Jeane (with an e).
She's a lovely lady, kind and sweet.
I'm lucky the Lord gave such a good sister to me.

She's been lots of places and done lots of things;
She's experienced both good health and bad.
But, she has come through it all with a smile on her face
And grateful for the blessings she's had.

Sometimes I know she feels really bad,
But she seldom, if ever, complains.
Her bravery (and stubbornness)
Must hide all her aches and pains.

She's a wonderful cook, and she makes pretty things.
Her house is a regular showplace.
She treats her pets as queens and kings
And her guests with the utmost grace.

If you could spend some time with Jeane,
You'd know these words are true.
If you never get a chance to do it,
I surely regret that for you.

I have three other sisters, three brothers too,
Each special in their own unique way.
But today I honor Jeane Malone,
My bright sunshine ray.

Poem by Alice Reed in honor of her sister, Jeane Malone, age 72, of Oklahoma City. Jeane spent many years living in various states and other countries including Okinawa and Thailand. In the United States, she worked in the banking industry. Her first diagnosis was at age 65, and the second was at age 68. Jeane has been part of a breast cancer trial study in order to help others. She is a mother of three children, a grandmother of eight, and a great-grandmother of two.

Her Legacy
Hazel Vail

Her joy was her family.
Her fear was to become a burden.
Her anger was the cancer.
Her grief was the loss of the breast.
Her laughter was in her smile.
Her healing was her positive view of life.

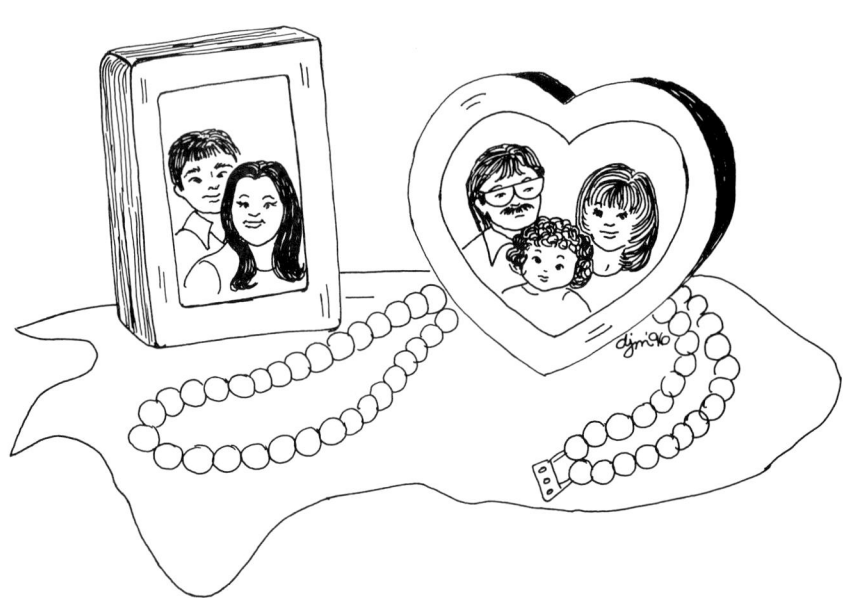

Submitted by Deborah Kifer in memory of her grandmother, Hazel Winfield Vail, of Kingston. Hazel, a housewife and employee at Tinker Air Force Base and Sears, was diagnosed at age 54 and died at age 70. A mother of five, grandmother of 21 and great-grandmother of 36, Hazel survived breast cancer for 17 years at a time when chemotherapy and radiation were virtually unheard of.

Main Ingredient: Delight
Christine Salmon

In 1964 when we first met as professor and student, her cancer had just emerged. For 20 years, Christine battled the disease in its varying forms with a bright eye, humor, and determination to live life fully.

I know so many people who also called Chris their mentor. Her teaching was rooted in her example. I marveled at her positiveness even in the face of cancer, and before I knew about the cancer, I delighted in her love of life. One sunny spring day as a ragtag bunch of us managed to make a late afternoon "Chris" class, she asked incredulously why we were there. After all, it was such a lovely day; she could not imagine that we would want to be inside when it was so wonderful outside. Of course, we were there because of her, to learn what she had to offer that day.

That day and many others through the years, she encouraged our sensuality about a world filled with beautiful things. To a long string of interior design principles such as balance, order, and rhythm, she added her own philosophy—delight. We learned that you should not design an interior that lacked delight as an ingredient. She taught a generosity of spirit and unflagging optimism. While she is my personal hero, her life and work also stand as monuments to an important woman in our history.

Christine: "Death is inevitable, you know. How you get from here to there is your choice."

Submitted in memory of Christine Salmon, of Stillwater, by Jan Jennings, her former student. Christine died at age 69, after being diagnosed at age 47. An architect, educator and public servant, Christine was the mayor of Stillwater, served as city commissioner, chair of the Stillwater Planning Commission, a member of the hospital board at Stillwater Medical Center, and was a partner in Salmon and Salmon Architects, specializing in the architectural needs of the disabled.

A Myriad of Memories
Jo Mott

Jo's cancer was inflammatory, but she never let her discouraging prognosis hinder her endeavors to care and support others, statewide (Oklahoma Breast Cancer Coalition) and nationwide (M.D. Anderson Support Network). She was a constant source of knowledge about breast cancer, cancer drugs, protocols, and surgery options. She often said, "I'll send you some information on that," and she always did, promptly.

Jo has now gone on to her new adventure, but she left behind her strength, perseverance, never-ending courage and a myriad of memories of one of the most dynamic, unique, beautiful people I have had the privilege to know. Her valiant fight is over, but her victories will live on to inspire us for many years.

Submitted by Beth Cronin, breast cancer survivor, in memory of her friend , Jo Mott, of Bethany, who died at age 54. Beth and Jo were fellow support group members of Promise at Mercy Health Center. Jo's initial diagnosis had been at age 50. A dedicated volunteer, her concern was always for others more than herself, and she had a phenomenal capacity for compassion and caring. In addition to PTA and other school functions, Jo worked diligently with the Breast Cancer Coalition to organize a letter-writing campaign to promote awareness of the need for increased funding for breast cancer research.

I Knew a Woman
Betty June Wheeler

I knew a woman
who used to plant periwinkles in her backyard.
She also grew roses;
her favorite one was a peach color.

I knew a woman
who would invite you over every Friday night
To eat spaghetti
and play dominoes 'til midnight.

I knew a woman
who came to live with me when I was about six.
She would put my hair up in a ponytail,
and we shared a big double bed.

I knew a woman
who found a small cyst.
Her doctor drained it and said it was nothing;
just watch it and see me again in six months.

I knew a woman
who died on Christmas Day.
Breast cancer had stolen her away.
I love you, Aunt Betty, and I'll see you over there.

Poem in memory of Betty June Wheeler, of Sand Springs, by her niece, Renita Taber. Betty died at the age of 44 after her initial diagnosis at age 42. She had been the assistant supervisor of the billing department in the Water Department for the City of Sand Springs for more than 20 years. She was married for 18 years, and was a devoted member of the Skyview Assembly of God for many years, serving as church treasurer for much of that time.

The Beach I Walked for You
Jennifer "Ginger" Morgan

Ginger Morgan lived through the long battle with breast cancer for six years, and each day she lived with zeal for life and determination to win. I met Ginger only three years prior to her death but the impact of her life and our friendship continues.

The only thing I ever heard Ginger say she wanted was to see the ocean. She didn't care which ocean; she just longed to dip her toes in the sandy water and listen to the sound of the waves. How I wanted that dream to come true for her. By the time we collected enough money for her to go, she was too ill, but she never let it get her down nor did she ever give up hope.

Once, while I was in Florida walking on the beach, I began to cry as I thought of Ginger. I couldn't understand why God would allow me to go where she had never been. So, I asked him for a big beautiful shell to take to her. In my dismay I went back to my room, then God began to give me answers to my questions through the following poem:

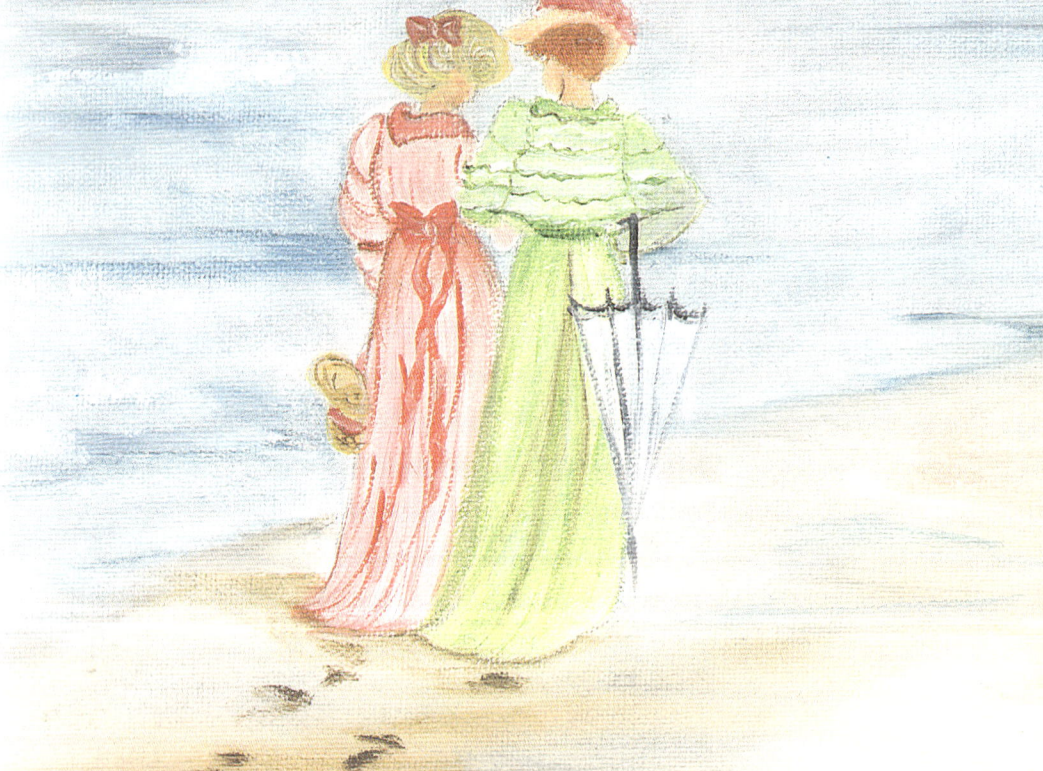

Preface and poem by Neta Archer in memory of her friend, Ginger Morgan, of Moore. Ginger was diagnosed at age 26, and died at age 32. She had been office manager of Leveridge Imports, and was a devoted daughter, wife, mother, family member, Christian, and friend. She worked hard to have a good marriage, and she did. She was also very active in the Southgate Elementary PTA, was a girl's T-ball coach, a Sunday school group leader and an enthusiastic volunteer. The painting, "The Beach I Walked for You," was done by another of Ginger's friends, Carol Nutty.

The Beach I Walked for You

Today I walked upon the beach
and I did it just for you.
I know you've had a great desire
to make this dream come true.

So as my toes buried deep
within the frosted sand,
I was reminded of your life
and spirit that is so grand.

I asked the Lord for a great shell
to bring to mind this day,
but He just gave me tiny shells
as I brushed the tears away.

I asked, "Oh Lord, where is the shell,
a grand one for my friend?"
He said, "Oh don't you understand
the small ones that I send

are all the beauty, love and joy
your sister has brought on earth.
She is a special, chosen one;
her life is of great worth."

So as I walked on down the beach,
I knew I had walked for you;
and some day we'll walk heaven's shores
where all our dreams come true.

But should you get there before me,
I'll meet you on the beach,
Where painless, perfect peace abounds
and all is within our reach.

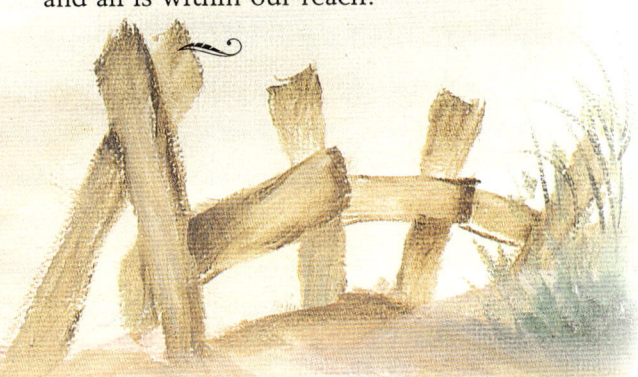

Poem by Neta Archer, friend of Ginger Morgan.

Carol Nutty

Meaning of Mothers and Daughters
Dorothy M. McAlister

In 1964, my mother and her college friend, Gwen, attended a convention in Wentworth By The Sea, New Hampshire. I was working in New York City at the World's Fair. We planned to meet in Boston after their meetings; the summer before, Mother had a radical mastectomy. This summer she had lots of energy. A week near the ocean seemed like a reward for healing so well.

After her meetings and a delicious prime rib dinner, Mother and I returned to our hotel room. After climbing into the double bed, she said she needed to tell me something. A heavy stillness filled the room. She had found another very small lump in her remaining breast. She had told the doctor that she would not consider surgery until this adventure to New England was completed.

I know I asked her how long she had been waiting to tell me. I guess she had planned to tell me in private. That was always her nature. The reality was that while she had been able to share it with me, giving it to me to carry, she could not shed it. It was hers. She apologized for leaving me this legacy. Oh God, what is the reason women continually say, "I'm sorry"?

The next day seemed lighter, perhaps because she had let go of her secret. She took us to a hardware manufacturing plant which produced materials she sold in her profession back in Oklahoma City. Then we drove to the Cathedral of the Pines in the mountains of New Hampshire, an outdoor sanctuary. As Gwen (whose own mother was facing death) and I marveled at the beauty, we held each other. We talked about the meaning of mothers and daughters and the reality of death. Mother rested in the car.

When they returned to Oklahoma, Mother's secret was more openly shared and she was able to carry the memories of surprise and delight. If she had died that summer, I think she would have felt her life very full. But she didn't die. She did have a second radical mastectomy, and she also lived to see four of her grandchildren born, lots more buildings go up and more hardware sold in her home city. At the time of her death in 1981, one of her sorority sisters wrote: "Dorothy's up in heaven checking out the hardware."

Submitted by Donna O'Keefe in memory of her mother, Dorothy McAlister, of Oklahoma City, who died at age 68. Donna, a chaplain at Oklahoma Medical Center, says her mother was initially diagnosed at age 50. Dorothy was business manager and vice president of McAlister Materials, a family-owned building specialties supply company. Her company furnished hardware, granite, limestone, windows, and doors for office buildings, hospitals, schools, and other commercial buildings. Dorothy's company also furnished the flag pole that is all that remains of the Alfred P. Murrah Federal Building which was bombed in Oklahoma City on April 19, 1995.

Ode to My Mother: Champion of the Door Slammers
Nancy L. Hane

A dungeon-sized smooth solid door

with a long black crack up the middle
Words echoing back, banging against the eardrums
"Go to your room, young lady,
and don't you come out until you're ready to apologize!"
No fat tender baked potatoes
No thick juicy steak
Just stale old gray musty cookies from the third grade
that were under the bed in a baggie
A flat glass of water in a green and white Dixie cup
A cardboard dinner
for someone with a cardboard brain
which cannot seem to absorb the fact that
you cannot win a fight with your mother.

Poem by Elizabeth Hane, daughter of Nancy Hane, age 50, of Norman. Nancy was diagnosed at age 35 when her daughter was 11 years old. Elizabeth was 16 when she wrote this poem, and is now 26 and working on her PhD at Brown University in Providence, RI. Nancy says that the tenacity of that little girl had something to do with her overcoming cancer.

Mother, Dear
Lea Ann Nowlin

I love my mother so
Although it sometimes doesn't show
She has never done anything to me
She has given me the best, you see
She doesn't deserve this mess
She says her faith is being put to the test
I can see on her face the fear
Yet she doesn't let out a tear

Poem by Alicia Nowlin, daughter of Lea Ann Nowlin, age 37, of Kingfisher. Alicia was 16 when this poem was written for her mother, who was diagnosed at age 35. Lea Ann has been married for 19 years and has two daughters. She is an employee of the Kingfisher County Conservation District, and a member of the First Baptist Church of Kingfisher.

Her Strength Gave Us Strength
Bettie Bernard

Bettie's son-in-law, Leroy, described her as "a stately and proud woman to whom family was Number One." She was a leader in the neighborhood as well, successfully coordinating all her activities—family, church, and profession. She always stood ready to help others as witnessed by her voluntary participation in the cancer research program at the Oklahoma Research Center, even when it was apparent she would not survive the battle. As she once said, "I hope my participation in the chemotherapy research will help to find a cure. This will keep others from pain and suffering and maybe from having to undergo deforming surgeries." As her daughter Bonnie put it, "It is important to know that her strength gave us strength which we all use today, encouraging other women regarding early detection, breast self-exams, mammograms, physician's exams, and education."

Submitted by Bonnie G. Kolar in memory of her mother, Bettie Bernard, of Oklahoma City, who died in 1969 at age 51. Bettie, who had been initially diagnosed at age 48, was a wife, mother, and office manager and administrative assistant for several hospitals in Oklahoma City. She was survived by her husband, three daughters, 11 grandchildren, and as years have passed, 12 great-grandchildren.

Our Model
Frances Searle Keesee

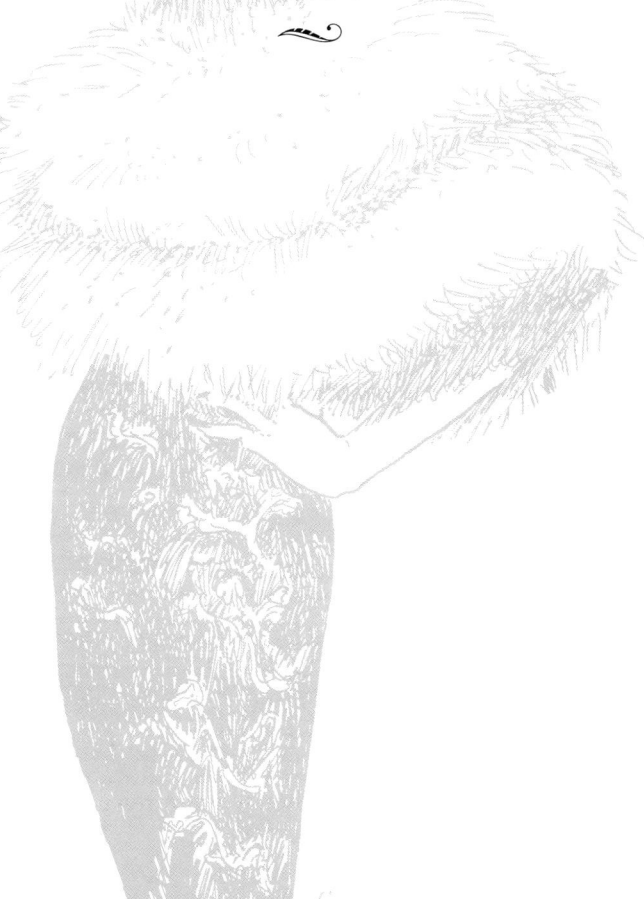

How ironic! Mom had changed our diapers many years ago; now it was our turn to help her get dressed, put on her lipstick, change her bedding, prepare her meals, pay her bills, give her medicine, hold her hand and encourage her. It seemed odd that our roles were now reversed. She taught us so much.

Mom had been a high fashion model, but she was in fact our role model! When cancer hit, the loss of her breast was devastating. But she kept on encouraging her friends and her children. It was her incredibly positive attitude that helped her defy the odds and live longer than any doctor had anticipated. Mom's zest for life touched everyone around her and is still a powerful memory.

Submitted by Liza Frampton and Becky Love, in memory of their mother, Frances Searle Keesee, of Oklahoma City, who died at age 52. Frances, a high fashion model, was diagnosed initially at age 45. She modeled in New York City, Honolulu and Oklahoma City. She was also a gifted pianist and entrepreneur. Her favorite work, however, was rearing her four children.

A Rainbow for My Mom
Gennie Johnson

Right now you are a rainbow reaching for the top
For the bright colors represent family and friends
who care and love you a lot!
Sometimes the road to 100% takes more than a day
But to help you with our love, support, and strength
your family and friends will be there all the way.
For you are young and strong
to regain complete health it won't be long.
To you Mother Dear the one we love
I wish you good health and happiness thanks to God above
So be determined, bountiful, and bold
You will win this battle
And at the end of this rainbow is your pot of gold
defined as 100% good health and happiness
and to keep you that way God will do his best.
I love you very much Mother Dear
your final outcome will be wonderful never fear
On this rainbow you must finish your climb
and you'll be well in no time!

Poem by Kelli Brook Johnson, daughter of Gennie Johnson, age 53, of Oklahoma City. Gennie was diagnosed at age 48, and her daughter knows that Gennie has never slowed down once during her battle with breast cancer. An active community volunteer, Gennie was most recently named to Leadership Oklahoma City in 1995.

The Rainbow of Achievement
Gennie Johnson

Now that you've reached the end of your rainbow
and successfully made it over the top
The colors representing family and friends
are still with you, non-stop!
You know the road to 100% took more than a day,
but all—willing to help you with our
Love, support, strength and hope—
we have been with you all the way.
You are still young and have shown
how strong you can be.
You are a winner, not a loser,
which is easy to see.
To the best Mother around,
who is loved so dearly,
You have achieved good health and happiness
we can all see that so clearly.
Thank you to God
for doing his part,
For He has been there with all of us
from the very start.
In this battle you have shown to be
determined, bountiful, and bold.
Now, you have reached the end of this rainbow
and are well deserving of your pot of gold
defined as 100% good health and happiness.
And to keep you that way,
your family, friends and God will do our best!
I love you very much Mother Dear!
Your final outcome is wonderful
No more fear!
On this rainbow
Now you have completed your climb
Only the best life can offer
Will be with you until the end of time!

Poem by Kelli Brook Johnson in honor of her mother, Gennie Johnson, July 2, 1991.

One Stone at a Time
Florence Brown

~~

If kindness and helping others were stones, my mother has built a mountain one stone at a time.

~~

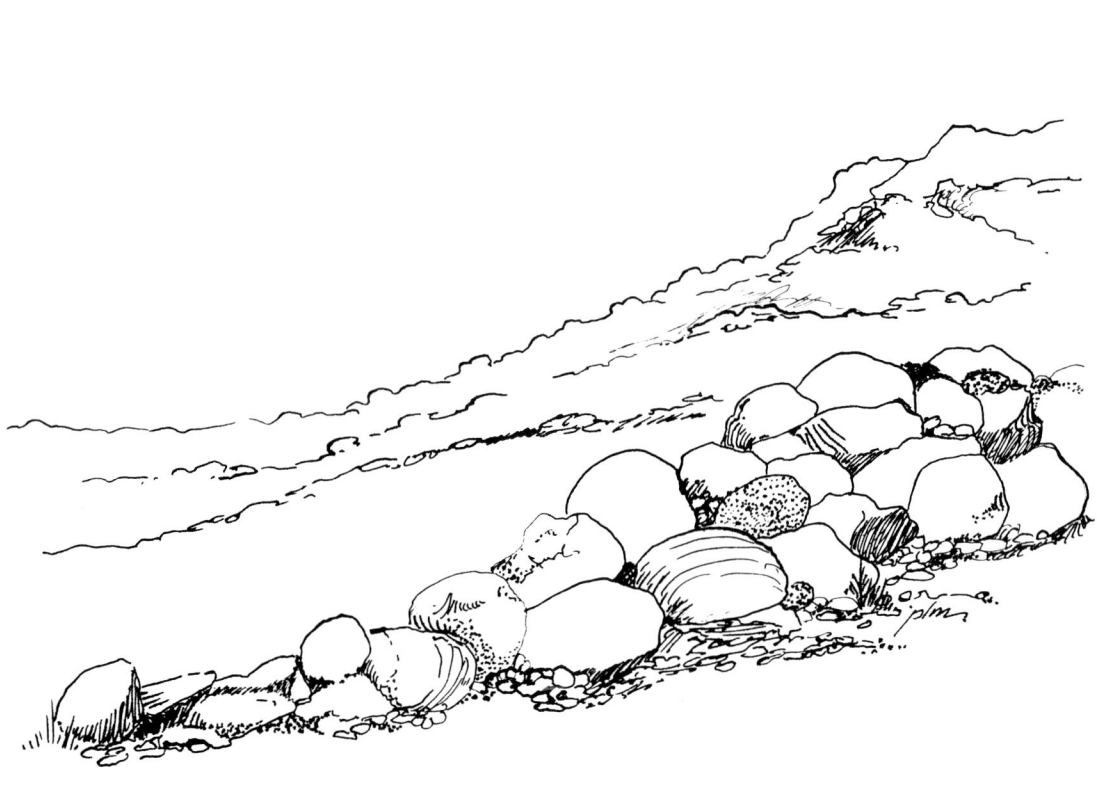

Florence Brown, age 83, of Elk City. Submitted by her daughter, Betty Stout. Florence was initially diagnosed at age 70. She and her husband farmed in the Leedey community before moving to Elk City in 1970 where she worked for Travelers Motor Club. She continues in this role today, and is active with the VFW Auxiliary and the American Legion Auxiliary, having held various offices through the years. Florence is also active in her church.

In Memory of Marcheta
Marcheta Long

She was a carpenter, plumber,
    mechanic, painter, and gardener
    but still had time to launder.

She planted and cared for shrubs, flowers, and trees,
    and it was not unusual to see her
    working on her knees.

She was very sympathetic for the sick and the old,
    but had no mercy for
    a gopher or a mole.

She was always busy and loved to cook;
    it seemed she never had time for
    a newspaper or book.

She was mother and friend to four daughters
    she brought into this life; and all through the years
    remained a loyal, dedicated wife.

She was called to Heaven on April 29, 1987.
    All her loved ones felt like lost fish
    in a big lake.

It was a time of bitterness, sadness, and fear;
    but we should all remember:
    God has never made a mistake.

Marcheta: "I apply the same line of thinking in dealing with cancer as when I am jogging—I don't look too far down the road as I might tend to get discouraged easily. I just concentrate on one little hill at a time."

Poem by Paul Long in memory of his wife, Marcheta "Keta" Long, of Choctaw. Keta was 46 when she died, having been diagnosed initially at the age of 42. She was a homemaker, wife and mother of four daughters. She played the piano for residents at several nursing homes, baked items for school and church functions. She was often "Mrs. Santa Claus" or the "Easter Bunny" at elementary school parties. Her philosophy was, "It's not the quantity of life which counts most, it's the quality."

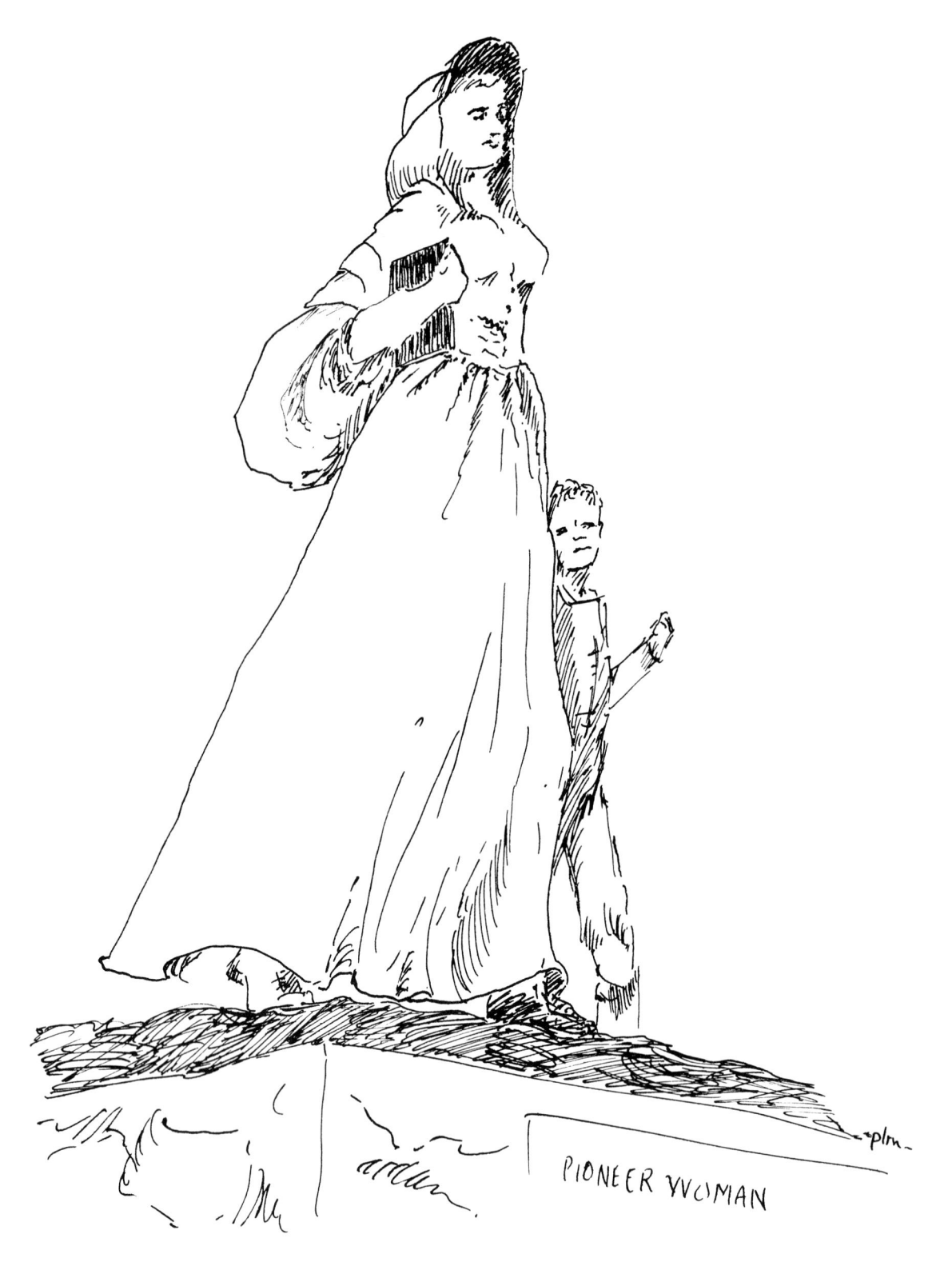

PIONEER WOMAN

Hero
Dianne Gumerson

Inspirational   Guiding light

Hero

Fighter   Loved life

Hero

Great example   Never felt sorry for herself

Hero

Grit   Determination

Hero

Valiant   Hopeful

Hero

Positive thinker   Courageous

Hero

Dianne Gumerson

Written by Gennie Johnson, friend of Dianne Gumerson of Oklahoma City. Dianne was initially diagnosed with breast cancer in January 1982, at age 38; her first recurrence was discovered in 1987; she battled metastases for nine years. Dianne died April 8, 1996, at age 52. The above words and phrases were used to describe Dianne by her Bosom Buddies, a cancer support group. We were all saddened by her death and shocked; she had bravely fought and endured the pain of this disease for 14 years. Her oncologist called Dianne "a true success." She was a miracle in the way she would come through so many crises. Dianne was and continues to be my "hero." Bill Gumerson, Dianne's husband and owner of Gumerson and Associates, was instrumental in assisting in the design and was responsible for the construction of A Portrait of Breast Cancer, *Phase I, the Pictorial Exhibit.*

Healing Energy
Betsy Crump

Those who knew Betsy Crump knew the intensity with which she lived her life, her art, and her relationships. She was passionately devoted to her work as a metal sculptor. A show at the Smithsonian Museum just after her first recurrence was, perhaps, her most remarkable artistic achievement. More importantly, it was the courage and determination she demonstrated in preparing her work despite the pain, the loss of strength and dexterity, and the discouragement caused by the recurrence of the breast cancer in her sternum.

Another of Betsy's remarkable characteristics was a talent for intentional living. She always gave so much of herself in everything to which she turned her interest. Somehow she had looked at the mysteries of life more deeply than most. Before her death in February 1993, she poured herself into the fight against breast cancer. The healing energy from her work, as she fought for her own life and against breast cancer as a woman's disease, gave her life new meaning and significance.

Betsy assumed leadership roles in the fight against cancer in her home county: she helped to establish a breast cancer support group at the hospital; she worked for the Breast Cancer Coalition to wrest more national resources; she left an endowment to the Oklahoma Make A Wish program to help support young persons with terminal diseases; and she was a driving force in the initial 24-hour Relay for Life for the Cleveland County (OK) Unit of the American Cancer Society. She was very proud to have recruited three teams. Today, the run's Spirit Award carries her name in honor of her work.

Betsy wrote the following poem the night of the April 1992 run.

Submitted by Rebecca Neathamer, best friend and caretaker, in memory of Betsy Crump, of Norman. Betsy died at age 38, following her initial diagnosis at age 34. Although breast cancer eventually was the cause of Betsy's death, cancer never conquered her. She lives on through the programs she helped found, and in the memories of her many friends who stood with her through the struggles.

Uncharted Journey
Betsy Crump

What strange sensations
sleeping out of doors in this tent
hearing the winds blow the sides and top.

Feels like I am on some type of vessel
that is moving through the wind
taking me on a new and uncharted journey.

And as I look at the night I see
a circle of luminaries
glowing in the dark.

Lights that remind me of those who have died
those still fighting
and those yet to be.

My wish is
that no one would ever get this disease again
it is just too hard.

I hope my breathing flying little dome home
takes me on a gentle trip
through the night.

And while I sleep
may I remember
those who are still walking throughout the night

Keeping vigil
Keeping watch
Keeping the hope glowing that some day
there will no longer be this disease.

Poem by Betsy Crump who died at age 38.

Acknowledgments

Project Woman™ gratefully acknowledges the following individuals, facilities, and corporations for their generous donations toward the publication of this book.

Project Woman Facility Donors

Central Oklahoma Chapter of the
Susan G. Komen Breast Cancer Foundation

Columbia Presbyterian Hospital

Deaconess Cancer Center

Diagnostic Radiology Imaging &
Breast Care Center

INTEGRIS Baptist Medical Center
Troy & Dollie Smith Cancer Center

INTEGRIS Southwest Medical Center
Southwest Breast Health Center

Mammography Center of Oklahoma
at MICO

Midwest City Regional Hospital
Renaissance Women's Center

Oklahoma Breast Care Center

Radiology Associates, Inc.

RGI-Radiology Group, Inc.

St. Anthony Hospital

University of Oklahoma Health Sciences
Center Institute for Breast Health

Friends of the Book

Lisbeth Alexander

BeautiControl

Cherokee Color Corporation

Lura Clark

Susan Deason

Isabel Fuller

Molly Griffis

Barbara Henderson

Susan Hogan

Grace Hollrah

Eleanor Irvin

Gennie Johnson

Ruth Lampton

Mary Jane McIlvain

Jean McKissack

McManus Litho Supply

Karen Pewthers-Yirak

Printers Bindery

Prisma Color Corporation

Resource Net

Stone Container Corporation

Walgreens Drug Stores

Kathy Williams

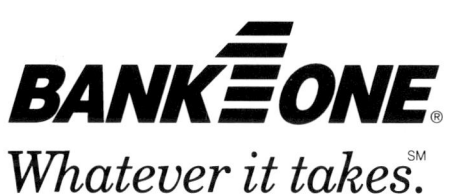

EXPRESSIONS IN WORDS AND ART

UNDERWRITERS

BANK ONE®

Whatever it takes.[SM]

Bank One, Oklahoma City
Member FDIC

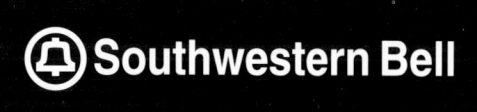

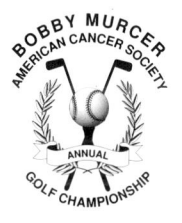

**The DeWayne Murcer
Memorial Foundation**

INTEGRIS Health[SM]

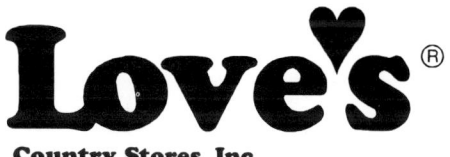

THE DAILY OKLAHOMAN

THE SUNDAY OKLAHOMAN

The Joullian Foundation, Inc.

An Anonymous Donor

Epilogue

In 1989, a remarkable event regarding breast cancer took place in the state of Oklahoma. A group was formed, an outgrowth of the American Cancer Society, which consisted of representatives from area hospitals, 17 breast cancer screening facilities, physicians, nurses, and medical administrators, the Oklahoma State Department of Health, the City/County Health Department, the Central Oklahoma Chapter of the Susan G. Komen Breast Cancer Foundation, the Oklahoma Foundation for Medical Quality, breast cancer survivors, and other citizens who wanted to volunteer their time and talents to provide broader education and awareness of the importance of early detection of breast cancer.

The formation of this group, which came to be called **Project Woman™,** was amazing in that all competitive walls came down between hospitals, screening facilities, and bureaucracies when the group held its first meeting. There were no hidden agendas; no secret plans to "outshine" a competitor. The mission was simple: "We must increase awareness and provide education to women regarding the importance of early detection of breast cancer, and to provide low- and no-cost mammography screening for women who cannot financially afford the examination."

For the past seven years, **Project Woman** has launched a major campaign each October during Breast Cancer Awareness Month. The campaign encourages Oklahoma women to make the commitment to get a mammogram, and participating hospitals and clinics are committed to provide discounted mammograms during that month. To date, **Project Woman** has received more than $60,000 to fund a no-cost mammography program for Oklahoma women who do not have the financial resources, through insurance or personal finances, to receive a mammogram. It is estimated there are at least 44,000 women who fit the American Cancer Society's risk profile who are financially unable to have a mammogram. In addition to the no-cost mammography, women screened through this program also receive a clinical breast exam and a Pap smear. We are beginning to make a difference. The no-cost mammography program is a joint effort of the American Cancer Society, the Oklahoma State Department of Health and of the Central Oklahoma Chapter of the Susan G. Komen Breast Cancer Foundation. The money raised so far has been funded through grants from the Komen's "Race for the Cure" events in 1994 and 1995.

Since 1993, **Project Woman** has sought to reach women through television news and feature stories of survivors and a "Take Charge" hotline phone for information regarding breast cancer. Fundraisers such as fashion shows and walk-a-thons have helped secure funding for our programs.

Then, in 1995, **Project Woman** conceived, developed and unveiled *A Portrait of Breast Cancer, Phase I,* an exhibition of photographic, literary and educational material. The photographic display portrays women from Oklahoma who have had breast cancer. Their faces represent our grandmothers, mothers, wives, sisters, and daughters. Some are no longer with us, but many of them have survived to tell their story. The display traveled across the state of Oklahoma, and returned in March of 1996 to the State Capitol Rotunda for the 1996

Legislative Session. The participants in the exhibit were honored by Oklahoma's First Lady, Cathy Keating, during a luncheon held at the Governor's Mansion. They also met with legislators to lobby for issues related to cancer. The exhibit continues to travel across our State to educate and raise awareness for our cause.

This book, *A Portrait of Breast Cancer: Expressions in Words and Art*, represents *Phase II* of the *Portrait of Breast Cancer* project. It reveals the stories and the artistic expressions of scores of women who have fought the battle. It is intended to be a tribute to any woman who confronts this disease. The book is the culmination of countless hours of dedicated volunteer work by a special group of women and men whose mission is to ensure that **Project Woman's** message will be heard.

Terry Gonsoulin

Terry Gonsoulin, Chair
Project Woman

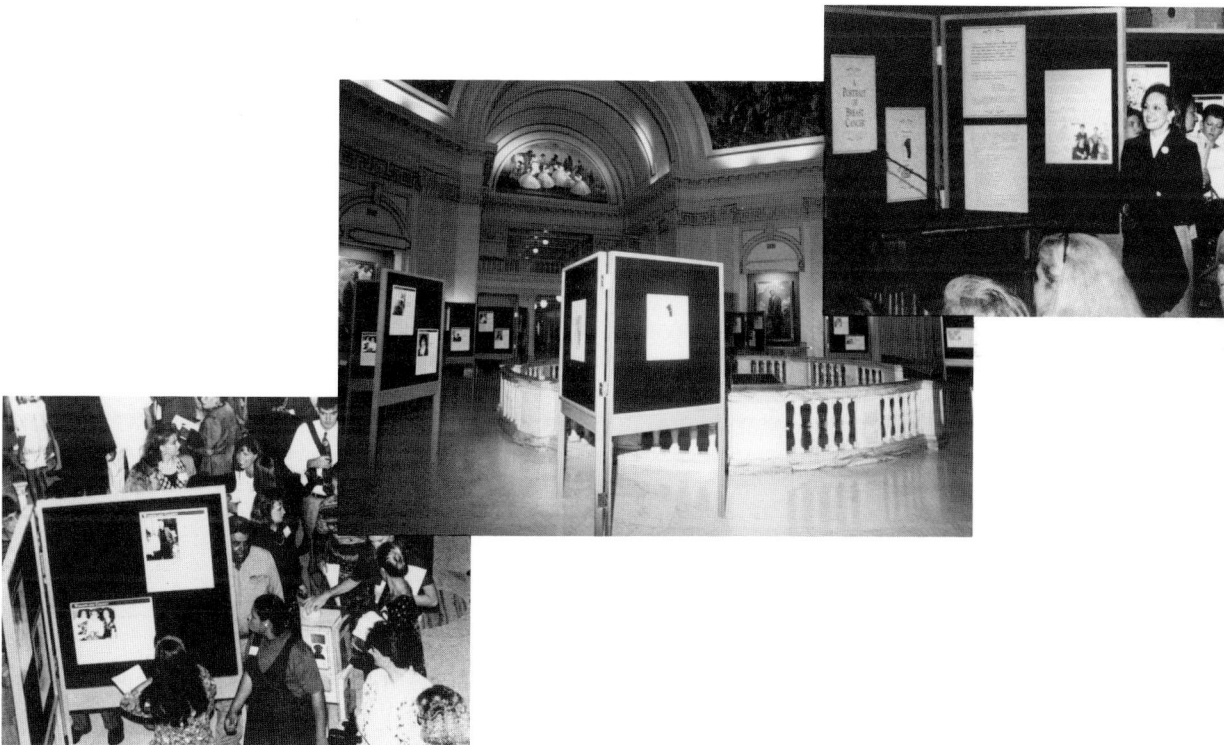

A Portrait of Breast Cancer, Phase I: A Pictorial Exhibit
displayed at Oklahoma State Capitol Rotunda, September 11, 1995

The Women of *A Portrait of Breast Cancer, Phase I*: A Pictorial Exhibit

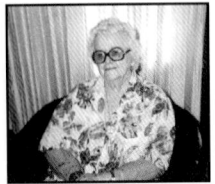
FLORENCE BROWN
BECKHAM CO.

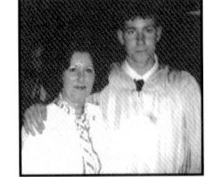
DONNA BECKER
BLAINE CO.

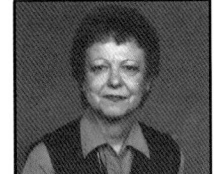
JERRY ANN ELMENHORST
CANADIAN CO.

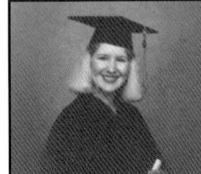
TAMMY MASS
CANADIAN CO.

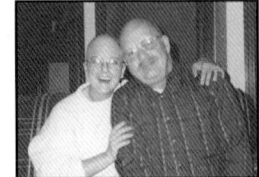
TRACY A. TURNER
CANADIAN CO.

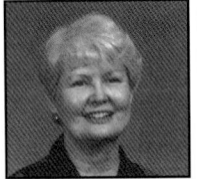
MARY PACE FALLING
CHEROKEE CO.

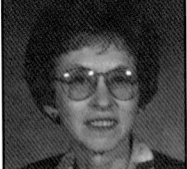
VERA FAYE WRIGHT
CIMARRON CO.

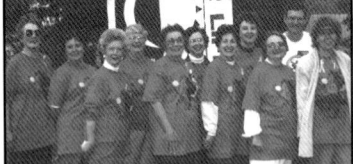
BREAST CANCER SUPPORT GROUP
RELAY FOR LIFE TEAM – CLEVELAND CO.

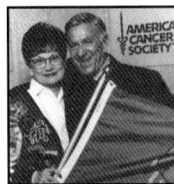
MARGARET L. LONG
CLEVELAND CO.

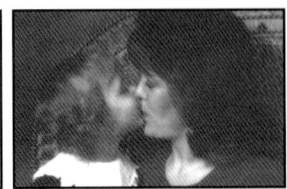
JENNIFER (GINGER) MORGAN
CLEVELAND CO.

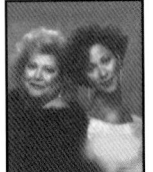
PEGGY JOYCE SMITH
CLEVELAND CO.

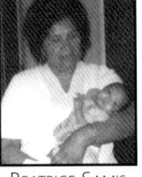
BEATRICE SAMIS
COMANCHE CO.

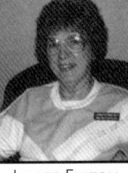
JANICE FULTON
CREEK CO.

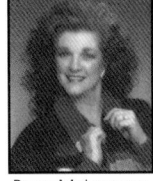
BETTY McLAUGHLIN
CREEK CO.

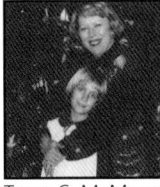
TEDDY C. McMILLON
CUSTER CO.

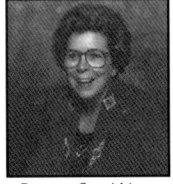
BOBBIE SUE WOLF
CUSTER CO.

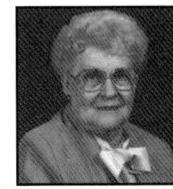
GRACE HOLLRAH
GARFIELD CO.

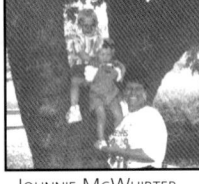
JOHNNIE McWHIRTER
GARVIN CO.

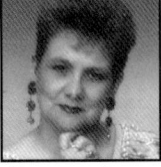
CHARLOTTA ATWELL
GRADY CO.

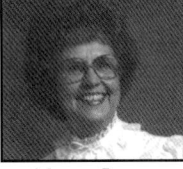
MARIAN EMBRY
GREER CO.

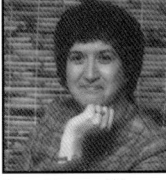
BETTY HOLMAN WHEELER
HUGHES CO.

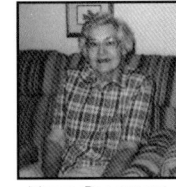
VERNA BLACKWELL
JACKSON CO.

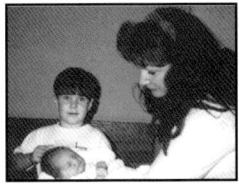
MARCIA MORGAN TOSEE
JEFFERSON CO.

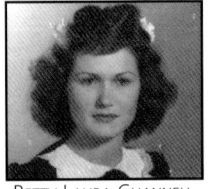
BETTY LAURA CHANNELL
JOHNSTON CO.

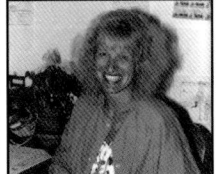
REBECCA SIMPSON
KAY CO.

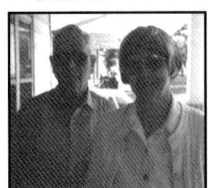
MURIEL E. WALLACE
KAY CO.

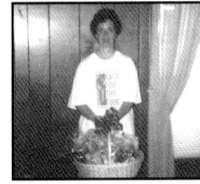
LEA ANN NOWLIN
KINGFISHER CO.

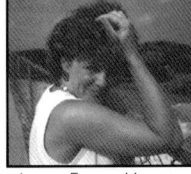
JOYCE ELAINE HOPSON
KIOWA CO.

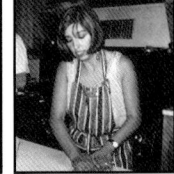
PATRICIA GUTIERREZ
HORNER – LEFLORE CO.

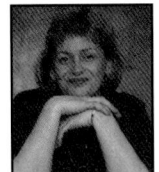
NINA RITCHIE
LEFLORE CO.

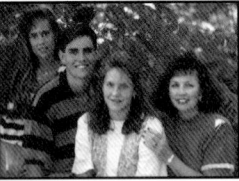
CAROL BOND PARKER
LOGAN CO.

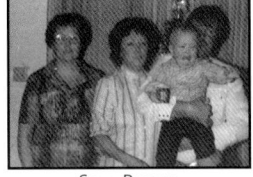
SIBYL BARBER
LOVE CO.

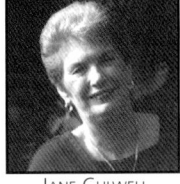
JANE CULWELL
LOVE CO.

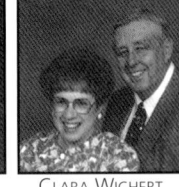
CLARA WICHERT
MAJOR CO.

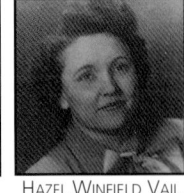
HAZEL WINFIELD VAIL
MARSHALL CO.

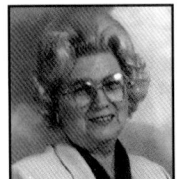
BETTY JANE BERGMAN
MAYES CO.

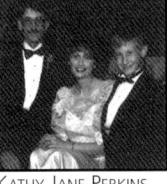
KATHY JANE PERKINS
MAYES CO.

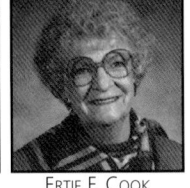
ERTIE F. COOK
McCLAIN CO.

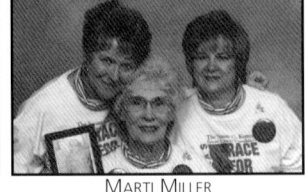
MARTI MILLER
McCURTAIN CO.

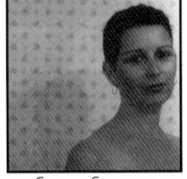
SUSAN SPENCER
McCURTAIN CO.

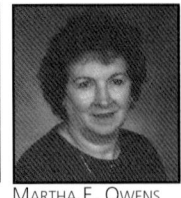
MARTHA E. OWENS
MUSKOGEE CO.

The Women of *A Portrait of Breast Cancer, Phase I*: A Pictorial Exhibit

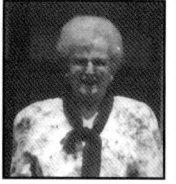
MARGARET SHIPLEY
MUSKOGEE CO.

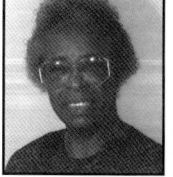
HELEN M. BROWN
OKLAHOMA CO.

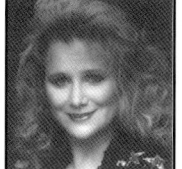
SHERRY ANN BRULE'
OKLAHOMA CO.

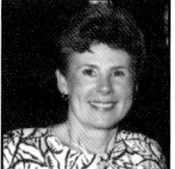
DIANNE GUMM GUMERSON
OKLAHOMA CO.

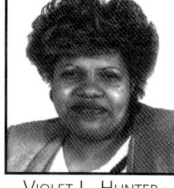
VIOLET L. HUNTER
OKLAHOMA CO.

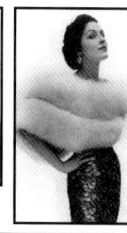

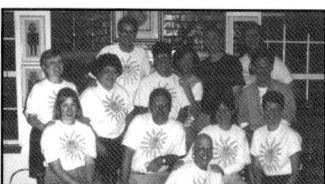
FRANCES SEARLE KEESEE
OKLAHOMA CO.

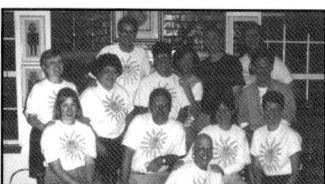
LINDA KIRKPATRICK
OKLAHOMA CO.

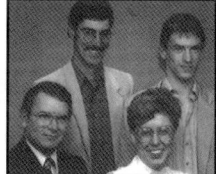
JO MOTT
OKLAHOMA CO.

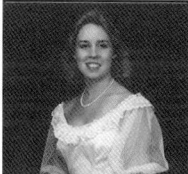
CARA RACKLEY
OKLAHOMA CO.

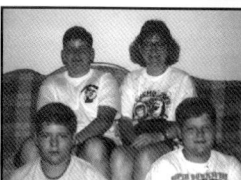
BETTY RAE MARSHALL
OSAGE CO.

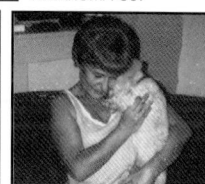
EILEEN STARLING
OTTAWA CO.

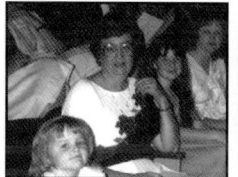
DORIS F. CALVERT
PAWNEE CO.

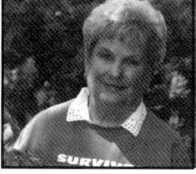
NORMA CODDING
PAYNE CO.

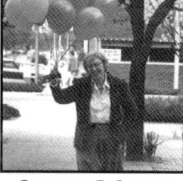
CHRISTINE F. SALMON
PAYNE CO.

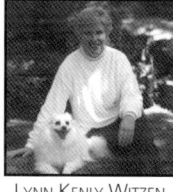
LYNN KENLY WITZEN
PAYNE CO.

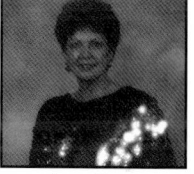
JEANE YATES
PAYNE CO.

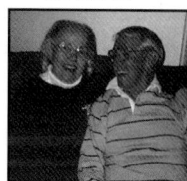
FRANKE M. RAYBURN
PITTSBURG CO.

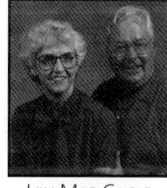
LILY MAE CAGLE
PONTOTOC CO.

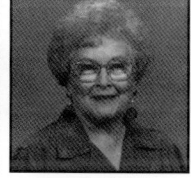
FERN M. PEERY
PONTOTOC CO.

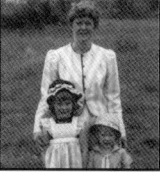
DEBORAH ANN GEE
PUSHMATAHA CO.

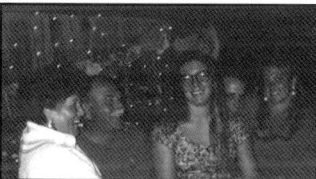
JACQUE COLLINS YOUNG
ROGERS CO.

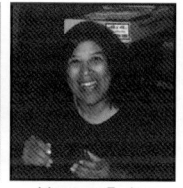
YVONNE E. JIM
SEMINOLE CO.

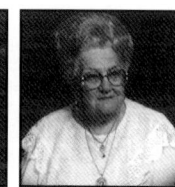
HELEN KUHN
STEPHENS CO.

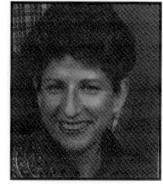
SUSAN LINDLEY
STEPHENS CO.

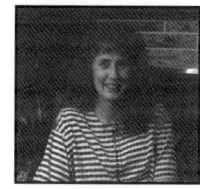
JODI LIESE
TEXAS CO.

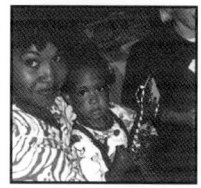
MAE LEWIS
TILLMAN CO.

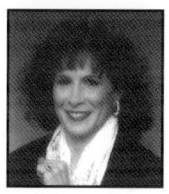
REBECCA DAY
TULSA CO.

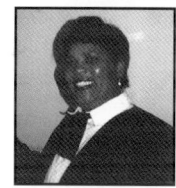
SANDRA EDWARDS
TULSA CO.

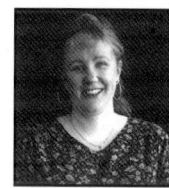
LISA A. EFAW
TULSA CO.

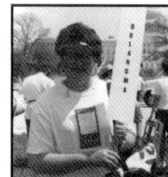
PEGGY L. FUNK
TULSA CO.

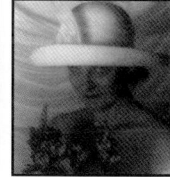
SHARON PETRIK
TULSA CO.

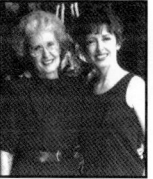
RUTH PRATT
TULSA CO.

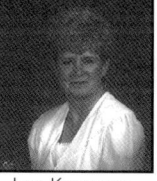
LOIS KENNEMER
WASHITA CO.

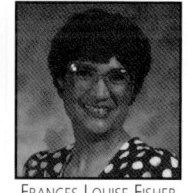
FRANCES LOUISE FISHER
WOODWARD CO.

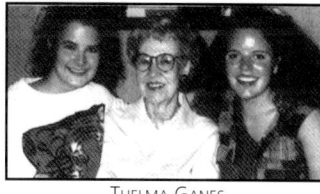
THELMA GANES
WOODWARD CO.

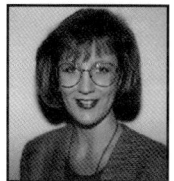
BETH SNIDER
WOODWARD CO.

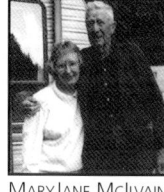
MARYJANE McILVAIN
WOODWARD CO.

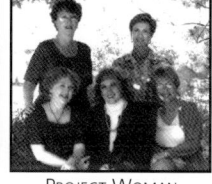
PROJECT WOMAN
COMMITTEE SURVIVORS

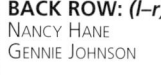

BACK ROW: *(l–r)*
NANCY HANE
GENNIE JOHNSON

FRONT ROW: *(l–r)*
PAT LYNN MOSES
TERRY GONSOULIN
ROSEANNA SMITH

179

Index of Honorees

Index of Honorees

Breast Cancer Screening Guidelines of the American Cancer Society

Mammography

By age 40, have a baseline mammogram

Age 40-49, every one to two years depending on mammography and physical findings

Age 50 and older, every year

Discuss with your health care professional any risk factors you may have to see if you should begin routine mammography at an earlier age.

Clinical Breast Examination

Have your breasts examined yearly by your health care professional.

Breast Self-Examination (BSE)

Starting by age 20 women should examine their breasts monthly. BSE is a good routine health habit that can help you know how your breasts feel normally. Any changes that are found should be reported to your health care professional. Remember, most breast lumps are not cancer. If you are having monthly periods, examine your breasts seven days after the start of your period. If you are no longer having periods, pick a day of the month that is easy to remember and examine your breasts on that day each month.

Follow these three steps when you examine your breasts:

1. In front of a mirror, look at your breasts with your arms raised overhead. Look for any change in the shape of your breast or in the skin. Then, rest your palms on your hips and press down firmly to flex your chest muscles. You should be looking for any change in shape, dimpling of the skin, changes in the nipple, or redness of the skin. Gently squeeze each nipple, looking for any unusual discharge.

2. Lie down and put a pillow or folded towel under your right shoulder. Place your right arm behind your head. Use the finger pads on your middle three fingers on your left hand to feel your right breast. Press firmly enough to know how your breast feels. Move around the breast in a set pattern. You can choose either the circle, the up and down line, or the wedge. Do it the same way every time. It will help you to make sure that you have gone over the entire breast area and to remember how your breast feels. Now examine your left breast the same way using your right hand. Remember to cover the entire breast area including under your arm. A firm ridge in the lower curve of each breast is normal.

3. Use this same examination pattern when you are in an upright position while in the shower or tub. Your hands will move over your wet skin making it easy to check how your breasts feel.

To order additional copies of

A Portrait of Breast Cancer

EXPRESSIONS IN WORDS AND ART

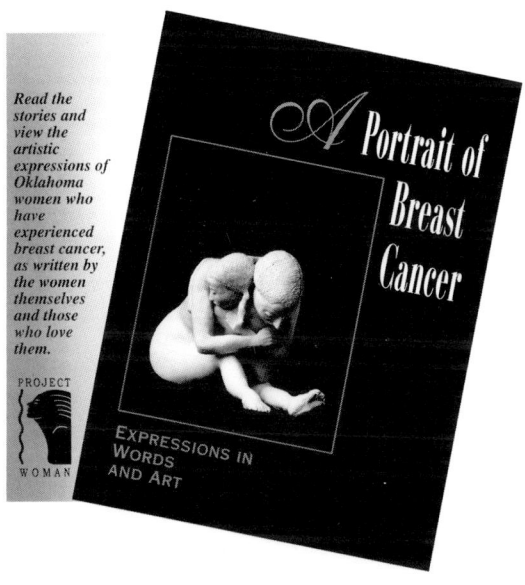

Read the stories and view the artistic expressions of Oklahoma women who have experienced breast cancer, as written by the women themselves and those who love them.

PROJECT WOMAN

Please send _____ softback copies of
A PORTRAIT OF BREAST CANCER
at the mail order price of $18.03 per book.
    Per softback copy . . . . .$12.95 plus
    Mailing cost 4.00
    Oklahoma tax 1.08*
    TOTAL $18.03

Please send _____ commemorative hard cover
copies of A PORTRAIT OF BREAST CANCER
at the mail order price of $31.59 per book.
    Per hard cover copy . . .$25.00 plus
    Mailing cost 4.50
    Oklahoma tax 2.09*
    TOTAL $31.59

* Oklahoma residents only

❏ Upon request: inscription in commemorative
copies only.
Inscription to read: (check one)
❏ In memory of

_____
(please print name for inscription)
❏ In honor of

_____
(please print name for inscription)
❏ Check or Money Order enclosed.
(payable to the American Cancer Society.)

❏ VISA ❏ Mastercard ❏ American Express

Card Number _____

Expiration Date _____

Signature _____

PROJECT WOMAN™

c/o The American Cancer Society
4323 NW 63rd Street
Suite 100
Oklahoma City, OK 73116
(405) 842-8829 or 1-800-733-9888

Proceeds from the sale of **A PORTRAIT
OF BREAST CANCER** will be used to
further the mission of *Project Woman,*
a committee of the American Cancer
Society.

Your Name _____ Total Amount: $ _____

Address _____ Phone (_____) _____

City _____ State _____ Zip _____

Please allow 4-6 weeks for delivery